MuscleAerobics™

The Ultimate Workout
For Body Shaping

Patricia Patano & Linette Savage
Foreword by Rafer Johnson

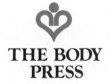

**THE BODY
PRESS**

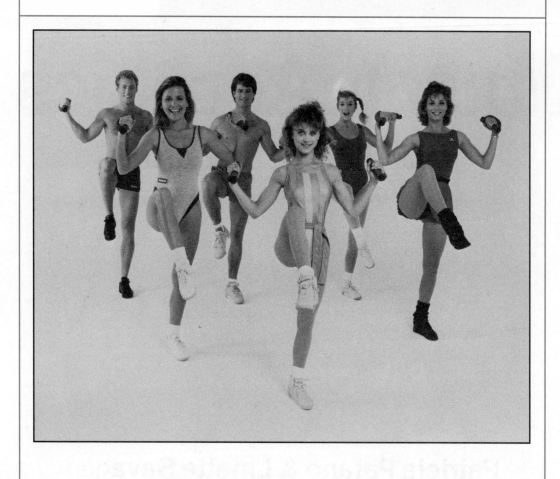

Published by The Body Press, a division of HPBooks, Inc.
P.O. Box 5367, Tucson, AZ 85703   602/888-2150
ISBN: 0-89586-361-8
Library of Congress Catalog No. 85-80118
© 1985 HPBooks, Inc., Patricia Patano and Linette Savage
Printed in U.S.A.

Publisher
Rick Bailey

Editorial Director
Theodore DiSante

Art Director
Don Burton

Book Design
Leslie Sinclair

Book Assembly
Paul Fitzgerald

Typography
Cindy Coatsworth,
Michelle Carter

Director of Manufacturing
Anthony B. Narducci

Photography
© 1985, Tim Mathiesen, Fuji
Photo Film. All rights
reserved by the photographer
and MuscleAerobics™

Hair Styling & Makeup
Dale Lawlor

Special Acknowledgments
AMF American Athletic
  Equipment
Fuji Photo Film U.S.A., Inc.
Reebok U.S.A. Limited, Inc.

Material prepared by
Rutledge Books, a division of
Sammis Publishing
Corporation, 122 E. 25th St.,
New York, NY 10010

Contents

About The Authors

Patricia Patano is a public relations expert who was most recently on the Los Angeles Olympic Organizing Committee (LAOOC) from 1981 to 1984 as Assistant Vice President of Public Relations. In this capacity, she was the liaison between LAOOC and all corporate sponsors. Before her term with the LAOOC, Ms. Patano worked in marketing and communications for Unitours/Club Universe, First Travel Corporation and Motel 6, Inc. She currently serves on the Board of the National Injury Prevention Foundation and the Los Angeles Boys & Girls Club.

Linette Savage is an Exercise Specialist who has studied aerobics, kinesiology, exercise physiology, anatomy and physical education. In addition to her duties as Finance Manager, she was also Fitness Director for the LAOOC during her four-year term. Ms. Savage is a recipient of the President's Council on Physical Fitness Award and is involved in many fitness organizations.

Together Ms. Patano and Ms. Savage have authored articles on fitness and are contributing editors of *Fit Magazine*. Together, they operate a modeling agency and marketing/promotion company specializing in fitness topics.

Dedication

We dedicate this book to our parents: Tom and Gladys Patano and in memory of Charles and Leticia Savage.

Foreword

As a gold medalist in the 1960 Olympic Games in Rome and as a torch bearer for the 1984 Olympic Games in Los Angeles, physical fitness has been, and always will be, a vital part of my life. A dedication to a lifestyle of health, fitness and athletics made these thrills possible.

Along the way, I've discovered that a few things are necessary to have a healthy lifestyle: It must be a commitment; it must be enjoyable; and it must be effective enough to really work.

Many people think of exercise programs as quick fixes that should do the job for you right away, with little effort. But neither life nor exercise is like that. Exercise is work, but it can be fun too. Getting and staying fit should be something we enjoy.

The exercise program in this book is just that. Yes, it requires dedication, but once you've made the commitment I think that you'll stick with it. You'll find that MuscleAerobics is an exciting way to get and stay in shape.

It works because it is a *total-body workout.* It offers a cardiovascular challenge you can live with. In addition, you exercise upper- and lower-body muscles to shape a better physique.

I've known the authors since our days on the Los Angeles Olympic Organizing Committee for the Summer 1984 Games. It is my pleasure to attest that their pursuit of excellence has been tireless, no matter what the task. This same attitude is part of the MuscleAerobics program they've created.

Being fit will contribute not only to your physical well-being. Your social, mental, emotional and spiritual sides will also benefit. So have fun and enjoy the new workout of the 1980s—MuscleAerobics!

Rafer Johnson
Gold Medalist, Decathlon
1960 Olympic Games, Rome

CHAPTER ONE

What Is Muscle-Aerobics?

We use the word *MuscleAerobics* to represent our complete aerobic-fitness plan. In MuscleAerobics you hold light weights in your hands while doing aerobic-type exercises. We consider MuscleAerobics a combination sport and weight program that you can do just about anywhere—at home, in an aerobics class or on a stationary bicycle.

WHAT IS AEROBICS?

Aerobics, or aerobic exercise, was coined in the early 1960s by Dr. Kenneth Cooper. His research showed that sustained cardiovascular exercise is a valid form of preventive medicine for maintaining general fitness. Cooper determined the cardiovascular and respiratory benefits yielded by different types of exercises. He then determined the minimum amount of "benefit points" one needs regularly to maintain health and improve fitness.

According to Cooper's research, you can get these points with *any type of cardiovascular exercise*—including running, walking, swimming and many other activities. Obviously, the critical part of an aerobics program is not necessarily the specific type of exercise. Sustained cardiovascular activity is the key to fitness.

He chose the word *aerobic*—meaning *with oxygen*—to represent this idea. Even so, the dynamics of the idea are more complicated than implied by the definition. Aerobics can be viewed as an intricate system of bodily supply and demand. That is, the body needs energy for any type of activity, and the need is filled by burning off the food we eat. Oxygen is the spark the fuel needs to burn.

Regardless, *aerobics* is the word in general use. The fact is that Cooper codified and organized what fitness means to many, many people. He is generally credited with being one of the main forces of the current fitness craze. The majority medical opinion is that aerobic programs strengthen heart muscle, increase the efficiency of lungs and offer other wonderful benefits.

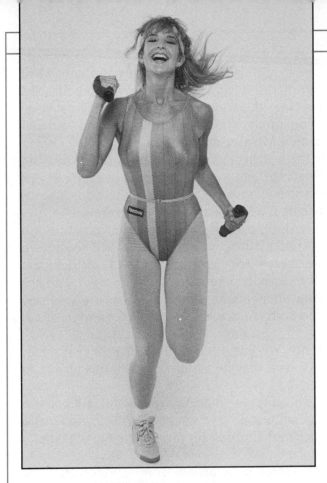

MuscleAerobics offers a total-body workout, using aerobic principles and light handweights, such as the AMF Heavyhands shown here.

WHY MUSCLEAEROBICS?

Our MuscleAerobics program is the perfect way to increase the benefits Cooper points out. In MuscleAerobics you hold handweights and move your arms while performing preferred aerobic exercises. This allows you to use both your upper and lower body. The net result is that you get the same aerobic benefits in less time than you normally gain using primarily your lower body. And, if you exercise for the same duration, the added weight gives you *more* aerobic benefit.

What Kind of Weights?—Don't confuse the handweights of MuscleAerobics with weights used in weight lifting. The latter is strictly a strength-building activity. MuscleAerobics is an *aerobic-exercise* activity. The weights you will use are light—from one to two pounds each. You use the light weights for a high number of repetitions.

This concept of light weights becomes even more effective when you use them in conjunction with leg movements. Though seemingly simple, the combination actually produces significant physiological benefits. And when you increase your speed and degree of movement, greater effects result.

What the Weights Also Do—The handweights will constantly test you. Most sports psychologists agree that no matter what the sport, the equipment used challenges the participant. In this case, the handweights offer additional *resistance* during motion. With them you improve muscular endurance and your cardiovascular system. You will become a MuscleAerobics "athlete."

Initially you might consider the weights cumbersome or burdensome. But the satisfaction you'll feel in mastering them will be rewarding in itself. As one sports psychologist has said, because equipment is not part of the man, it needs getting accustomed to before it becomes an integral part of the exercise.

Once you've made the MuscleAerobics decision, a continuing program will make the added weight merely second nature. The handweights will become an essential part of your exercise gear—just as sneakers and clothes are. Eventually, you'll find it difficult to imagine exercising without them. Perhaps you'll even feel unprepared without them. Once you adapt to MuscleAerobics, you'll be amazed at your advanced performance levels when exercising without handweights.

Why MuscleAerobics Is Different—We know that you've seen or read other aerobic-exercise and sports books. You may be wondering why this plan is so special and different. Here's why:

Current "fitness fanatics" are hungry—some famished—for athletic adventure. Many fitness and sports enthusiasts have sampled tennis, racquetball, aerobic dancing and other activities in their quest for physical and psychological "self-mastery."

Lack of time has probably prevented most people from seriously pursuing any of these sports on a daily or regular basis. The result is that too few take time to include weekday fitness in their lifestyle. At best, you become a "weekend athlete." At worst, you exercise even less regularly, if at all.

The fact is that the true adventure in fitness is not just the sports we play or the fitness activities we do. The adventure comes from better everyday health and an improved self-image.

MuscleAerobics satisfies the common frustration experienced by those who want fitness but don't have two hours a day for a total-body workout. Done regularly during the week, MuscleAerobics will enhance your weekend sports performance. MuscleAerobics may not necessarily make you better in your particular sport—only consistent practice will help you do that. But it *will* get your body in condition to play the sport.

The popularity of aerobics has led experts to devise new methods for achieving even greater all-around fitness. Doing just aerobics conditions the heart and lungs and offers weight control. MuscleAerobics is better because it offers all that and more! With MuscleAerobics you work and condition both your upper and lower body at the same time. It is the ultimate workout.

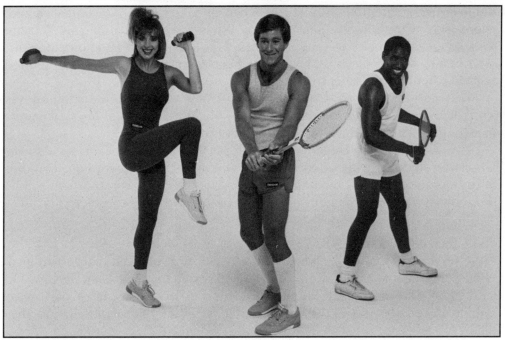

MuscleAerobics is not just a great training program. You can think of MuscleAerobics as a sport, too. It improves fitness and coordination and offers special challenges and goals. In MuscleAerobics, however, you "compete" only against yourself.

PRESENT TRENDS

Increasing awareness about fitness is a trend on the rise, becoming more pervasive daily. For some, it can dictate how they spend money and time. You've probably seen quite a few health clubs and exercise studios in your city. And if your city is like ours, Los Angeles, you'll often find health clubs, dance studios and exercise studios all on one street! Every major-city magazine and newspaper prints a list of the popular exercise and health clubs in the city. And virtually every major department store in the country has added a special department carrying fitness equipment.

Studies also show that cigarette smoking and alcohol consumption are on the decline. Many people are trying to eat less red meat and more chicken and fish. Refined sugar and white flour are being substituted with less-processed products in home-cooking.

And it doesn't stop there. New research and studies are being conducted to provide up-to-the minute information on health, exercise and performance improvement. Go to a magazine stand and count how many health, fitness and sports magazines are available. Check your daily newspaper for the Health Section. There's bound to be one there.

People are always looking for better ways to get in shape, to lose weight and to challenge themselves. Look what happened to jogging. The initial competitions were marathons for elite runners. When the general public felt left out because they couldn't run long distances, 5-kilometer and 10-kilometer runs, jog-a-thons, walk-a-thons and wheel-a-thons were introduced. They allowed everyone, not just the elite, to participate.

But the fitness fanatics still weren't satisfied, and the ultramarathon was born. Now we have the Ironman Triathlon, the ultimate test of physical endurance for the 1980s, a decade of competitive fitness.

In a way, the same thing happened to aerobic dance and exercise. Perhaps MuscleAerobics is to aerobics as the triathlon is to the marathon. In other words, aerobics is good, but MuscleAerobics is the next best step. You will be amazed to discover the benefits of a daily, one-hour MuscleAerobics workout.

PSYCHOLOGICAL BENEFITS

Everyone wants to be and stay fit, but not everyone can realize that goal. What some people lack is sufficiently strong motivation to stay healthy. Or, motivation may be intense at first and then gradually lessen. What causes people involved in regular fitness or athletic programs to quit before they achieve their goals?

Studies suggest that childhood experiences separate the self-motivated person from the rest. For example, if your parents instilled the value of sports and exercise in you, they are probably second nature to you. But if participation

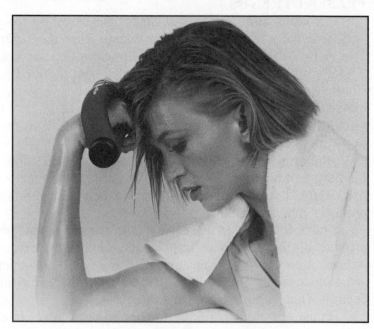

The benefits you'll gain from MuscleAerobics are many—not the least of which is the psychological benefit of feeling better about yourself.

in health and fitness was not emphasized as you were growing up, then keeping yourself healthy and trim doesn't come naturally.

Burnout—Once you've solved the motivation problem, you may discover another—called *burnout.* It is a condition produced by working too hard for too long in a high-pressure situation. It is accompanied by a progressive loss of energy and purpose.

This may sound like something experienced only by top athletes. Not true! Any time a sport or fitness program no longer creates personal satisfaction, you are subject to physical or psychological burnout.

The psychological aspect of sports has influenced many women in their feeling about exercise. Until recently, women were discouraged from sports or exerting themselves physically at all. This, of course, resulted in a lack of enjoyment of sports. Consequently, women have a harder time sticking with it.

The right sport, however, is the answer. The prospect of better health and weight loss are good motivators; MuscleAerobics contributes to both areas. Your increased sense of self-worth as you become more fit will help you keep going once the program is underway.

By working out the MuscleAerobics way for any length of time, you'll start to think of yourself a little differently. You'll become more active, more energetic and more athletic. An attractive self-image is difficult to give up. As long as you enjoy what you're doing, you're very likely to continue doing it. We think that will be the case once you start MuscleAerobics.

THE MUSCLEAEROBICS PROGRAM

MuscleAerobics imposes no age, sex, size or endurance limitations on its participants. It combines muscular fitness with cardiovascular techniques that take you through a warmup stage, mild exertion, greater exertion and then a cooling-down period.

MuscleAerobics has enough diverse movements so you won't collapse of boredom before you tire physically. We've created sports-related MuscleAerobics exercises that mimic movements from existing sports, including aerobic dance. In addition, you set your own pace and your own goals, according to your ability and interest.

MuscleAerobics will give you the best of everything—a workout for the heart plus flexibility and strengthening of major muscle groups. And, most important, it fulfills the basic requirements of any effective exercise program: *overload* by submitting your muscles to a task beyond the normal limits of your ability; *progression* by adding additional weights; and a *regular exercise program* performed at least three, but preferably five, times per week.

What It Feels Like—Now that we've given you all the positive arguments supporting a MuscleAerobics program, let's create a *feeling* of MuscleAerobics. Get a pair of one-pound dumbbells or similar weights.

If you don't have any dumbbells or handweights available, find an item that weighs approximately one pound and fits easily in your hand. For example, try a couple of wrenches from the tool chest.

Next, put on some upbeat music and walk around the room pumping your arms over your head to the beat. What do you feel? Now, pick up the pace to a slow jog and pump your arms high in front of you. How do you feel? What kind of sensations do you feel in your arms? How's your breathing? You walk around all the time and rarely feel out of breath. You can get an idea of how much harder your lungs and heart have to work when you add just a couple of pounds.

By sustaining this activity for at least 15 minutes, you can experience the type of workout you get from MuscleAerobics. Research demonstrates that you must physically "stress" your body beyond comfort to improve your aerobic fitness level.

About This Book

We cannot hope to cover the huge body of exercise knowledge within the confines of one book. Rather, we intend to convey the excitement and satisfaction you can get from one regular exercise program that works.

As you proceed with it, you'll eventually understand the vital concepts of a lifestyle embracing exercise and fitness. You'll get the physiological and psychological benefits you want—and perhaps need.

Before describing exercises, we cover some history behind the use of light weights. But if you are in a hurry to get exercising, skip ahead to chapters 3 and 4. In them we explore the meaning of an aerobics program and discuss the self-evaluation you should do before starting. In remaining chapters, you learn the MuscleAerobics program and how to customize it to fit your needs.

CHAPTER TWO

History Of The Dumbbell

Lifting heavy objects for competition or show probably dates back millenia. It's easy to picture prehistoric men trying to outdo each other lifting heavy rocks. Early cave drawings don't give us a clear picture as to the emphasis man placed on strength, but Biblical history certainly does. You only need read about David, Goliath, Samson and Daniel to know that strength and health were considered important.

As we continue to reflect on ancient history, we might even classify the Egyptians as the ultimate weightlifters due to their daily "training" regimen as the Pyramids were built. Imagine a daily workout involving moving stone after stone—2,300,000 per pyramid—each weighing approximately 2-1/2 tons. That's not unlike a group of people lifting Oldsmobiles all day long!

ORIGINS OF THE DUMBBELL

You can't study the history of exercise and fitness and ignore the role that weights—particularly *dumbbells*—have played. Dumbbells as an exercise tool have their roots in Ancient Greece. A special kind of dumbbell was used as extra weight for athletes competing in the long jump in the ancient Olympic Games. The unusual shape of these early dumbbells allowed the weight to be easily held. This ancient implement became the predecessor of the modern dumbbell. In many ways it bears a remarkable similarity to some of the grip weights currently made by various manufacturers.

19th-Century "Gymnastics" — There's little other recorded history of the dumbbell before the 19th century. During the 1800s, a variety of gymnastics programs were developed. They incorporated the new concept called *calisthenics,* coming from the Greek words *kalos,* meaning *beautiful,* and *athenos,* meaning *strength.*

This "beautiful strength" was enhanced by drills with wands and dumbbells. Dumbbell drills performed to music soon became not only a popular form of exercise but a political tool as well. In 1807 a German named Freidrich Ludwig John, considered to be the father of exercise programs, led large numbers of youngsters in group gymnastics both for physical enhancement and to inspire patriotism.

These popular gymnastic festivals, called *Turnfests,* were used to rally people around various political causes, drawing large crowds of devoted exercisers. Turnfest events became an international trend and stayed popular well into the 1900s. The dumbbell drill was a major activity, and many physical-education journals of the time published the new exercises presented at many Turnfests.

One Turnfest reported in the *San Francisco Chronicle* in 1915 featured the attendance of hundreds of people from 11 cities. The dumbbell exercises were similar in many ways to the MuscleAerobics exercises coming up in chapter 6.

FROM TURNFESTS TO TODAY

The drills of the Turnfests, though not very cardiovascular in nature, were really the predecessors of MuscleAerobics and many of today's aerobic exercise classes. The drills were set to music and followed specific patterns. The exercises consisted of body and weight movements. Turnfest exercise programs were rather intricate with directions such as "Step left forward and raise bells forward — 1, 2, 3, 4 count. Bend left knee and move bells sideward — 5, 6, 7, 8."

Early "MuscleAerobics" Researchers — Another remarkable aspect of the Turnfest was the active participation by women. In Dr. Dio Lewis's book, *The New Gymnastics for Men, Women and Children* published in 1862, he includes drawings of women swinging two- to three-pound dumbbells in a series of exercises. The clothing worn by these women resembles an exaggerated layered look — a far cry from skintight exercise clothes currently in favor.

The discovery of the correlation of upper-body activity and cardiovascular fitness had its roots during the late 1800s. Robert J. Roberts, a founding father of the YMCA, observed that if exercise with weights were done quickly it "brings heart and lungs into strong action."

In 1862, Dr. Dio Lewis not only touted the benefits of "strength, grace, flexibility, agility and endurance," resulting from using light dumbbells, but he also found that "a complete, equable circulation of the blood is thereby most perfectly secured." He called it "the superiority of light gymnastics."

Had someone just performed these dumbbell drills while running in place for 20 minutes, MuscleAerobics would have been created at the turn of the century!

In 1896, Dr. William Gilbert Anderson dedicated a chapter in his book *Methods of Teaching Gymnastics* to the "Use of Light Apparatus." He focused on the results of total-body workout by using lightweight dumbbells. An imbalanced musculature was of great concern to Anderson.

He realized that the hard-working farmer of his time was not immune to "one-sided" development and would benefit from the use of lightweight dumbbells. "No man stands up straight and mows," wrote Anderson of the farmer. "When he shovels, he bends more yet . . . plowing is better for the upper body; but it does not last long . . . chopping is good for the upper man; but does little for his legs." In this way the farmer was making some parts of his body strong and leaving others weak. Balanced strength and overall conditioning were the focus of Anderson's message.

Waning of Dumbbells—The extremely popular use of lightweight dumbbells diminished considerably in the 1920s and 1930s. Despite the decline, however, use of gymnastics-type dumbbells were found onboard the Queen Mary in the 1930s as part of the elaborate exercise equipment in a gym for first-class passengers.

Succeeding generations used heavier weights as an aid in bodybuilding or strength training. And there was a definite shift from calisthenics to more concentrated sports activity.

The 1930s brought the concept of play and recreation to full bloom in physical-education programs in schools. Dumbbell drills were replaced with sports such as football, basketball, volleyball and swimming. Training for these sports meant playing them. It appears that common-sense notions of balanced strength, popular in the late 1800s, were ignored as old-fashioned.

Unfortunately, a focus on total-body development was replaced by interest in less active "country-club" sports such as golf, tennis and recreational swimming. People became weekend athletes, playing sports to get in shape instead of getting in shape to play a sport. Increasing urbanization meant that more people sat while working. Obesity was becoming a trend, and the farmer was now seen as the prime example of physical fitness.

Post-War Years—Many articles published in the 1950s point to a less active lifestyle—*How You Can Exercise Without Moving*, *Reduce by Improving Your Posture* and *Stretch for a Good Figure* are three notable examples. By this time the spare tire and midriff bulge were receiving considerable attention.

It all led to the 1960s version of fitness—the American starvation program called the *diet!* Thin was in, at all costs. We drank water, ate grapefruit and overdosed on bran, carrots and tuna. Finally the great desperation to be thin exposed

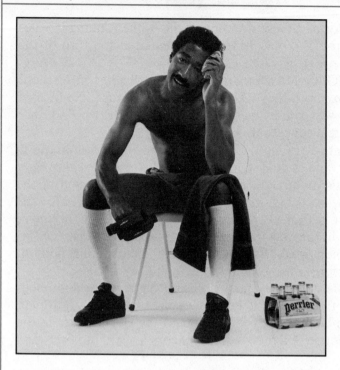

We guarantee that MuscleAerobics will give you a great workout. You'll "work" toward improved flexibility, muscle tone and endurance.

the horrors of *anorexia nervosa* and *bulimia*.

Modern Trends—The 1970s and 1980s have been more sensible. They've seen a return to common sense and a rebirth of "fitness means work." Exercise helps make the impossible, possible. Benjamin Franklin said it all: "Mankind mistake(s) difficulties for impossibilities. This is often the chief difference between those who succeed and those who do not."

A body weakened by diets and lack of exercise constantly *demands*. The message of today, however, is that the body *obeys* when constantly improved by regular exercise programs like MuscleAerobics. You *can* gain a semblance of control over the process of aging. Our bodies are wonderful creations that respond to positive input.

Even though most modern dumbbells are heavy and used for bodybuilding and strength training, the popularity of programs like MuscleAerobics have changed people's minds about using weights. MuscleAerobics and similar programs are "reinventing" the programs of the late 1800s that emphasized muscular endurance and balanced development.

Modern sports medicine and exercise physiology indicate the benefits of such programs. We're glad that MuscleAerobics is part of this rediscovery. The popular exercise program of the 1880s becomes the updated total-body conditioning of the 1980s—MuscleAerobics!

CHAPTER THREE

About Muscles And Aerobics

Fit to be Tied read the catchy title of an article printed in the *Los Angeles Times* of November 21, 1984. Jack LaLanne, at age 70 called "the flamboyant grandfather of the American physical fitness movement," swam one mile towing 70 boats with 70 people aboard, with his hands and feet bound. He did all of this in two hours and 25 minutes! "When you get the mind and body working together, you can do anything," said LaLanne.

Although we wouldn't recommend that you try this extraordinary feat, it certainly is an amazing display of a lifetime's involvement in a well-rounded fitness program. Jack LaLanne demonstrated mind and body working together. But he was also exhibiting remarkable muscular strength and superb cardiovascular conditioning, or in more general terms, muscle and aerobics.

We're not saying that MuscleAerobics is a program to set you down the stream with 70 boats tied to your back. But it is a program that will help you meet personal fitness goals.

In this chapter, we specifically define the basics of both muscle and aerobics. By looking at each component relative to the whole program, you'll understand what MuscleAerobics is all about.

As mentioned earlier, MuscleAerobics advocates the use of lightweight dumbbells or handweights—one to two pounds—in an aerobics-class setting or on a stationary bicycle. MuscleAerobics is beneficial because the added resistance of the weights during these activities markedly increases muscular endurance and oxygen capacity.

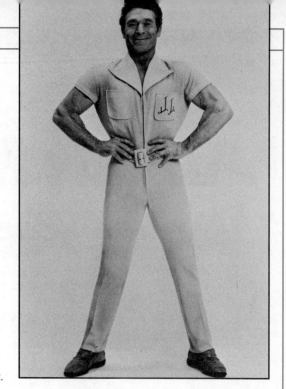

As Jack LaLanne proves, age is no barrier to fitness. You are never too old to get and stay in shape. MuscleAerobics is a great place to start.

You'll be able to reach beyond the current levels you are experiencing in your aerobics class because you will be further developing upper and lower body. Most aerobic sports limit activity to the lower body. Consider running, cycling and walking. All can be greatly enhanced by also activating the upper body. Our program takes these sports further and uses the total body.

The rest of this chapter uses a question-and-answer format. It's an easy way to settle any of the uncertainties you may have about muscles and aerobics. We aim to convince you that you've made the right choice with MuscleAerobics.

WHY DO I WANT MUSCLES?

They were tall, attractive and in the best of shape. At the end of the 19th century, they were known all over the world because of their unbelievable power and feats of strength. Although they were women, they had bulging biceps and rippling muscles. These "mighty Amazons of the stage" were called Athleta, Vulcana and Sandwina. And they were all women!

But you probably remember only the legendary Charles Atlas who claimed the title of the world's most perfectly developed male. Male or female, these "bicepian beauties" had one thing in common: well-developed muscles.

When we think of *muscles*, we tend to imagine huge bodybuilders with massive strength packed into a bronzed body. Don't worry, MuscleAerobics *will not* make you a bodybuilder. And the type of strength MuscleAerobics offers *will not* produce massive muscles all over your body. Furthermore, if you previously could not lift a piano, you still won't be able to. What MuscleAerobics will help you produce is *muscle tone, shape* and *endurance.*

Regardless of your present level of fitness, you already have a lot of muscle. Muscles make up nearly 40% of your total body mass. At rest, their energy requirement and oxygen needs are extremely low. But during heavy exercise, 90% of the blood leaving the heart is directed to the muscles.

Bones form the body's framework. Muscles protect it and allow it to move freely. Stop to think about it—muscular action is involved in more ways than we realize. Communication involves the use of our facial muscles. Whenever we blink an eye, it involves the muscles in our eyelid. Any study of the human body will eventually focus on the body in motion—muscles and their action.

WHAT IS MUSCLE?

Muscle comes from the Latin word, *musculus,* which literally means *little mouse.* The word developed from the appearance of certain muscles. When you consider that some bodybuilders have biceps measuring 23 inches around, it *can* look like there might be some mice in there.

People vary greatly in size, shape and structure, and so do muscles. Muscles

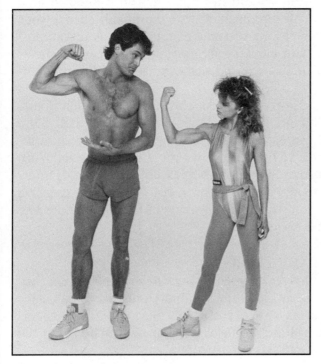

Women's muscles don't develop like a man's. In addition, MuscleAerobics offers better muscle tone, not more bulk.

are basically collections of cells called *muscle fibers.* The arrangement of fibers within a muscle is referred to as *muscle architecture.* An individual's muscle architecture determines how strong and how big a muscle actually gets.

Hundreds of individual fibers make up one entire muscle. These fibers are classified into two major types—*fast-twitch,* or *white-muscle,* and *slow-twitch,* or *red-muscle.* Large muscles of the body can contain many thousands of each type of muscle fiber.

People who are involved in high-endurance sports, such as triathletes and marathon runners, have a good supply of muscle fibers that seem to never tire—the slow-twitch type. For example, Julie Moss, winner in the women's division of the 1982 Hawaii Ironman Triathlon, probably has more slow-twitch fibers than fast-twitch fibers. But don't take this term to mean that she is slow. Everytime you use your muscles, you charge or "fire" them. Slow-twitch fibers fire at a slow rate, so they don't tire easily.

Someone like Olympic sprinter Evelyn Ashford is loaded with fast-twitch fibers. These fire rapidly but also tire rapidly.

We won't burden you with details about fast- and slow-twitch fibers—when and how they are activated. But you should know that the *amount* of slow- or fast-twitch fibers you have is genetically determined. For example, if you were born with 80% slow-twitch muscle fibers and 20% fast-twitch muscle fibers, you would grow old with the same distribution. If you wanted to be a competitive sprinter with that muscle composition, you'd probably change your mind eventually. You'd be better at long-distance events, such as marathons. Your muscle fibers would allow you greater success running longer distances. This explains why two people of similar size and shape can acquire different athletic skills.

If you are curious about your own balance of slow- and fast-twitch fibers, there is a way to determine it. Dr. David Costill, a scientist at Ball State University, Indiana, developed a muscle-biopsy technique. The procedure involves using a steel-shafted needle to remove from a muscle a grain-sized piece of tissue. Although this doesn't sound like a pleasant experience, it yields interesting results about cell structure and composition. If you want an inexpensive and painless alternative, experiment with various sports or fitness activities and try to determine what you do best.

WHAT TYPES OF MUSCLES ARE THERE?

Muscles can be divided into two categories—*voluntary* and *involuntary.* When you exercise, you tend to be aware of the voluntary muscles you use. For example, when you lift your arms above your head during MuscleAerobic exercises, you are aware of the voluntary muscles in your upper body. At the same time, however, involuntary muscles are in action.

Heart-pumping is an example of involuntary muscle action. It is interesting to note, however, that while the heart is an involuntary muscle, it is composed of muscle tissue similar to our voluntary muscles, which are thicker and stronger.

A thorough review of anatomy soon leads to the discovery of other muscles that act involuntarily. Without any effort on your part, the walls of your arteries, which are composed of muscle cells, expand and contract. So do the walls of your stomach and intestines. Other muscles in your body that do not operate under the control of your will are located in your lungs, gall bladder, kidneys, windpipe and a good many other places.

WHAT ARE SOME VOLUNTARY MUSCLES?

Starting from the top and working down, excluding facial muscles, the main muscle groups are: *trapezius, pectoralis, deltoids, triceps, biceps, latissimus dorsi, rectus abdominus* (abdominals), *obliques* (waist), *iliopsoas* (hip flexors), *gluteus maximus* (buttocks), *quadratus femoris* (quadriceps), *bicep femoris* (hamstrings), *tibialis anticus* (shins), *gastrocnemius and soleus* (calf) and *achilles* (heel).

If you refer to the muscles shown on pages 22 and 23, you can see where these muscles are located. The words in parentheses above are the common names used to identify them.

HOW MANY MUSCLES DO I HAVE?

There are more than 650 muscles in your body. This number holds true whether you are a 5-foot, 98-pound female ballerina or a 6-foot, 250-pound linebacker.

In addition, it *is* possible to work all of the voluntary muscles. But when you consider that your face has more than 35 muscles, it is not likely that you would work them all with any degree of concentration.

WHICH MUSCLES DO I USE DURING MUSCLEAEROBICS?

To discuss all the muscles involved would take a long time. And besides, it's not necessary for you to learn all of them for your daily exercise. However, we will discuss the major muscles controlling a number of common exercise movements. Refer to the photos on the next two pages.

Lower Leg—The muscle group used in foot movement and placement during walking and running is the *tibialis anticus,* next to the shins. Flex your foot up and you'll feel the muscle tighten between knee and ankle.

Pointing your toes down uses two muscles that form the calf on the back side of your lower leg. These are called the *soleus* and *gastrocnemius.* These mus-

MUSCLEAEROBICS ANATOMY LESSON

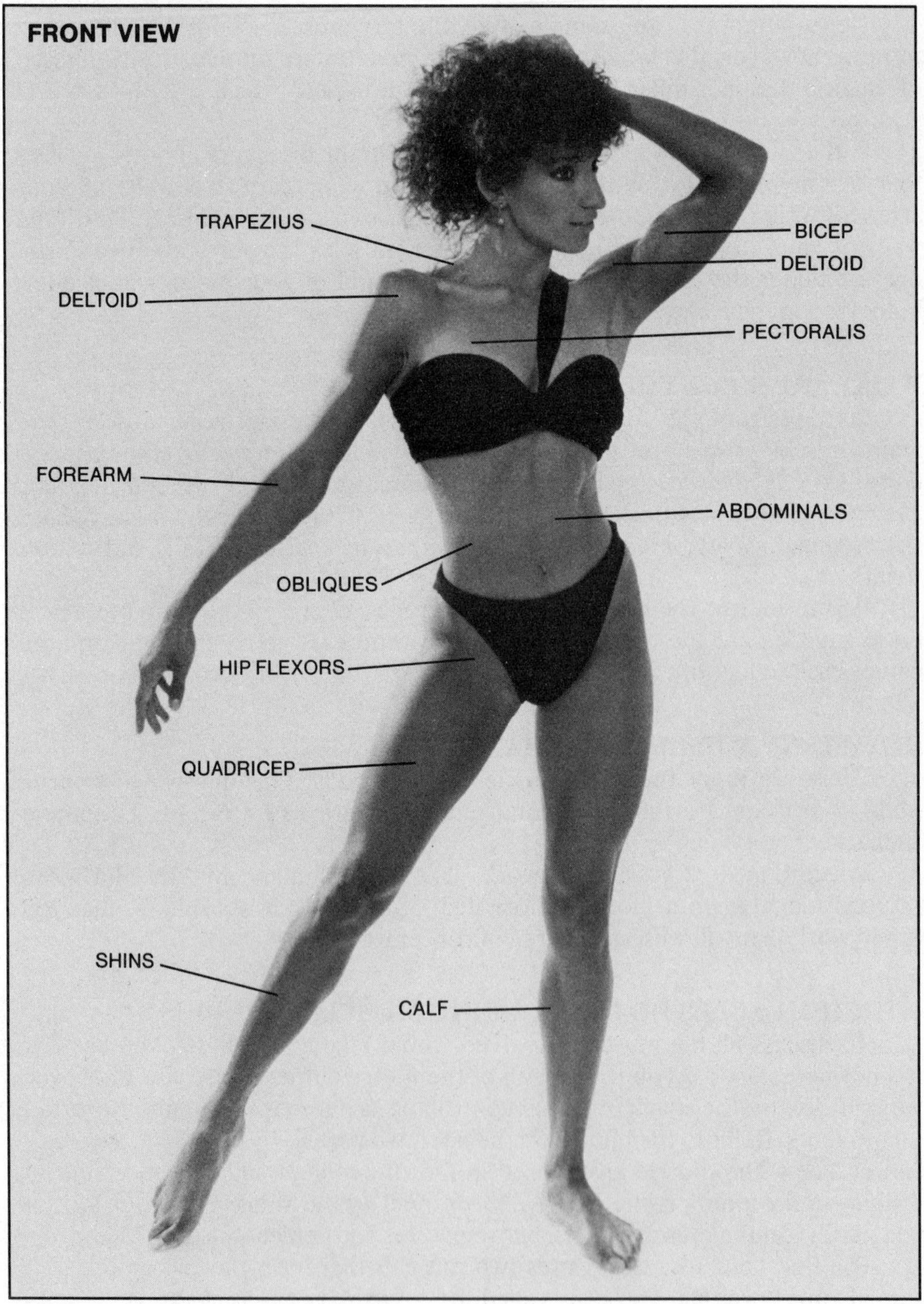

FRONT VIEW

TRAPEZIUS

BICEP

DELTOID

DELTOID

PECTORALIS

FOREARM

ABDOMINALS

OBLIQUES

HIP FLEXORS

QUADRICEP

SHINS

CALF

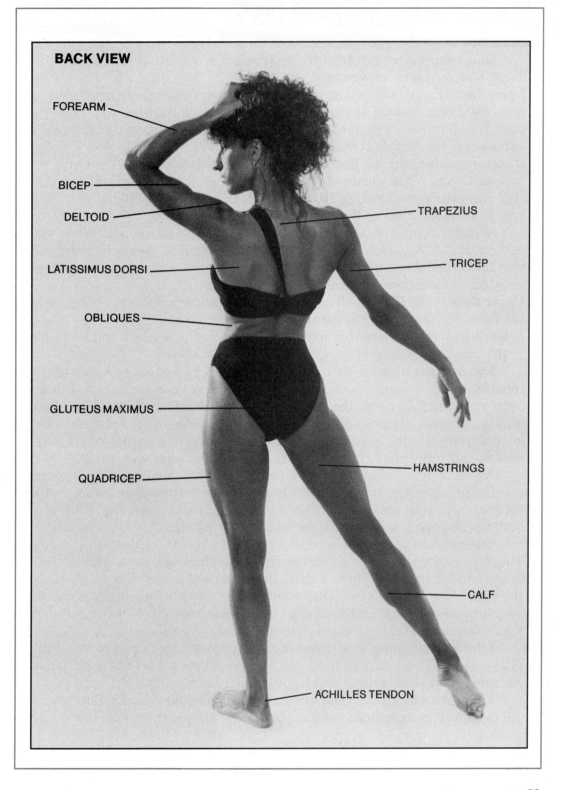

BACK VIEW

FOREARM

BICEP

DELTOID

LATISSIMUS DORSI

OBLIQUES

GLUTEUS MAXIMUS

QUADRICEP

TRAPEZIUS

TRICEP

HAMSTRINGS

CALF

ACHILLES TENDON

23

cles can be used differently, depending on the speed of foot movement.

Your knee joints support all the bodyweight above them during many different MuscleAerobic movements.

Upper Leg—Every time you extend the knee when running, it is controlled by your *quadriceps,* located at the front of your thigh. Everytime you bend the knee, it is controlled by your hamstrings located on the backside of your thigh.

Torso—Any bending movement at your hip joint is contributed by your *iliopsoas* group of muscles, the hip flexors. These are located deep within the lower abdominal cavity. When you do situps with bent knees, your hip flexors come into play. Any activity requiring you to lift your thigh high or forcefully, such as high knee lifts, will develop hip flexors.

Abdominal muscles run from your pelvis upward to the ribs. When you perform MuscleAerobics, the up and down movement of your arms combined with the up and down movement of your legs create a balanced toning of your stomach, or more correctly, your abdominal muscles.

Upper Body—The upper body begins at your shoulder girdle. On the right and left sides of your shoulder girdle are shoulder joints, commonly referred to as a *ball-and-socket joint.* Upward-lifting movements with the arms are made possible by the shoulder girdle.

The *trapezius* muscles, in the upper back, aid in controlling many of the shoulder-girdle movements. For example, pumping your arms up and down over your head involves the mobility of your shoulder girdle, upper-back muscles, shoulder muscles and upper-arm muscles. Also included in shoulder joint movement is the large *deltoid* muscle. It covers your shoulder joint. Everytime you lift your arms to the side, deltoid muscles becomes active.

Any activity in which your arms pull *toward* your body, such as a rowing movement, develops *latissimus dorsi* muscles. These large muscles are in the upper sides of your back. Any activity in which your arms push *away* from your body develops *pectoralis* muscles, the muscles of your chest.

During the many upper-body movements performed during MuscleAerobics, the muscles of the shoulder, chest and back interact with other, smaller muscles. These include the *biceps* and *triceps.* The *triceps* are at the back of your upper arm. They control your elbow joint when you extend your arms. Any movement requiring you to bend your elbow is controlled by your *biceps,* located at the front of your upper arm.

Muscles controlling wrist, hand and finger movements are in your forearm or lower arm. These muscles have long tendons crossing wrist and finger joints. Because you will hold a handweight, you'll use these muscles.

MuscleAerobics is designed to benefit your voluntary muscles. But remember that involuntary muscles, such as your heart, will greatly benefit, too.

WHY DOES MUSCLEAEROBICS HELP MY MUSCLES?

The motions and resistance in MuscleAerobics cause the muscles to help move blood, waste products and other body fluids throughout the body. MuscleAerobics creates dramatic changes in the muscle fibers and also increases the number of *capillaries* that supply blood to our muscle tissues.

Capillaries are the smallest blood vessels in which oxygen transfer occurs. They operate in the lungs, at the beginning of the oxygen cycle, and at the end of the cycle when they deliver oxygen to the muscle cells. Capillaries are also channels for the exchange of water and nutrients. Capillaries reflect the activity level of the muscles. In other words, MuscleAerobics increases not only our supply of oxygen-enriched blood, but also the number of capillaries delivering the blood to our muscles.

WILL MUSCLEAEROBICS MAKE MY MUSCLES BULKIER?

No, but you can improve muscle tone and shape. In proportion to weight and size, women's muscles are weaker than men's as shown on page 19. As a rule, women's muscles have approximately half the strength of their male counterparts. Muscular strength is related to the size and anatomy of the body and is indicated in terms of its proportionate mass—approximately 43% in males and 36% in females.

This is the result of endocrine function during puberty. It creates the fundamental sex differences in weight and development. The testosterone hormone in males produces a marked increase in the enlargement of muscle fibers. Female hormones have a growth-inhibiting effect. This automatic regulation means that women's muscles can be developed only in relation to their hormonal levels.

MuscleAerobics will condition your muscles, giving muscular endurance, thereby making you stronger. Muscles are your main source of power. They cause movement, and they also allow you to change the movement of your body. Strong muscles are able to produce more force than weak muscles, but you don't have to develop large muscles to become significantly stronger.

After performing MuscleAerobics for a few months, you won't be able to press a 100-pound barbell. But you will be in better physical shape to carry on daily activities with less effort.

How Muscle Tone Develops—As you recall, muscles are made of fibers. When tension or resistance is applied to a muscle, the muscle involved usually hardens and bulges. This is commonly called *contraction,* or *shortening,* of the muscle.

The opposite movement is *relaxation* of the muscle, or *releasing the tension.* In this case, the muscle lengthens. To visualize this idea, bend your arm at the elbow and make a muscle in your *bicep.* This contracts the muscle. See how it bulges and how the bicep appears to be "balled up" and shortened. Now,

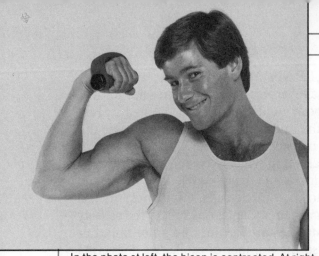
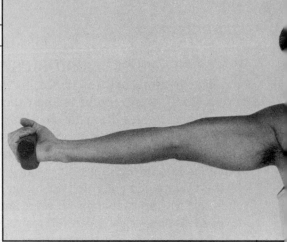

In the photo at left, the bicep is contracted. At right, it is relaxed.

straighten your arm and see the bicep relax and lengthen.

When a muscle contracts under normal conditions, only a portion of its fibers is used. By adding resistance—such as weight—you activate more fibers, eventually resulting in a stronger and firmer you. When performing arm work in an aerobics class without weights, you use a small portion of your muscle fibers. The muscle is not used to its fullest potential. By adding some weight in a MuscleAerobics program, you automatically activate more muscle fibers, and this leads to more strength.

How Muscles Are Shaped—Because MuscleAerobics makes you use more muscle fibers than usual, some muscles will get *slightly* bigger. But, we must add that, in general, many repetitions with light weights *do not* produce bulky muscles in *either* men or women.

The weights you use for aerobic benefits during MuscleAerobics are not the same as those you'd use if training for a bodybuilding contest. Aerobic weights usually weigh between one and five pounds. These small weights will produce *muscular endurance,* which creates lean, toned muscles—not muscular bulk.

Adding weight or resistance to your upper body activates more muscle fibers—something that doesn't happen in normal everyday use. The extra weight in your hand will help you become stronger and develop muscle tone at a much faster rate.

WHAT IS PROPER MUSCLE MOVEMENT?

To simplify our anatomy lesson, assume that the skeletal-muscular system consists of two bones with a joint between. them. One muscle flexes and another extends the joint. In reality, your body consists of joints at your shoulders, elbows, knees and so forth. Our bones act as supports and levers. Human movement is the result of the interaction of two types of forces—the external force or gravity and the internal forces controlled by your muscles.

Bones are connected at joints. These permit a variety of movements when muscles crossing them contract. In other words, muscle movement is determined by joint movement. When you move a part of your body in its normal direction, as in bending a knee in, it is called *joint flexion.*

When you move your knee from the flexed or bent position to its starting position, it is called an *extension* of your knee joint. For example, stand as your starting position. If you bend a knee, you're flexing it. When you return the foot to the floor, you've extended the joint.

Now, let's continue with your starting, standing position. When you bend all the way forward from the waist, you are flexing at your hip joint. If you return to your upright position, you are creating a hip extension. But if you keep extending, you would almost be do a back bend. Any extension movement that continues *past* its starting position is called *hyperextending.*

Other movements are *rotational,* or twisting, movements. These can be best explained with a foot. Rolling a foot inward is called *pronation.* Rolling the foot outward is called *supination.* You're probably most familiar with the rotational or twisting movements performed at the waist or hip joint.

In MuscleAerobics you restrict movements to the proper direction of the joint. Hyperextension is not correct. It goes against the natural design of your joints and can lead to injury of the joints or surrounding muscles.

WHAT OTHER FACTORS PLAY A ROLE
IN MUSCLE DEVELOPMENT?

Muscles are the primary force in movement. But joints, which are held in place by *ligaments* and *tendons,* help determine the range of movement. As just explained, bones meet with each other at junctions called joints. The structure of the joint determines how a muscle moves. A muscle's position and how its attachment crosses a joint will also determine joint movement.

Muscles attach to the bone via tendons. Ligaments help hold the bones together at the joints. Unlike muscles, ligaments do not have the ability to contract. They are not as pliable as muscles. However, both ligaments and tendons are similarly affected by physical activity because they function together.

Research studies that examined rats before and after training show the effects of training on ligaments and tendons. According to Dr. Richard A. Berger, physical training tends to increase the strength of tendons and ligaments and their attachments to bone. This enables them to withstand more stress within a wide range of movements.

CAN MUSCLEAEROBICS HELP ME BE MORE COORDINATED?

Understanding how your muscles move will give you increased body awareness, which leads to improved coordination. Coordination is a necessary part of any sport or exercise program

Think of coordination as the working of various muscles to create harmonious movement. In some cases the movement is predetermined, such as a new dance step. In other cases, the movement is unpredictable, such as when you must quickly respond to an unexpected set of circumstances. Coordination—or the lack of it—can be obvious. Remember the last time you tripped over something? A quick, coordinated reaction kept you on your feet and helped you avoid injury.

Coordination is necessary even when standing, walking or waving hello. Coordination skills are developed as we move from infancy through childhood and on to adulthood. These motor skills involve to a great degree our muscular development. The more we are in control of our muscles, the quicker our appropriate response, making us more coordinated.

MuscleAerobics generates muscular action over your entire body. This means that several large muscle groups are working harmoniously—in coordination. Because MuscleAerobics also works to build strength and endurance, your muscles respond by working, moving and reacting with greater efficiency. This type of activity helps to develop better coordination because the muscles have been subjected to various types of movement.

The seemingly insignificant addition of a one-pound handweight when performing MuscleAerobics will build strength. Also, the many repetitions performed during MuscleAerobics will generate muscle endurance. It is a combination of strength and endurance that improves coordination. A dancer has coordination, not because she has simply learned the movement, but because she also has strength to perform the step.

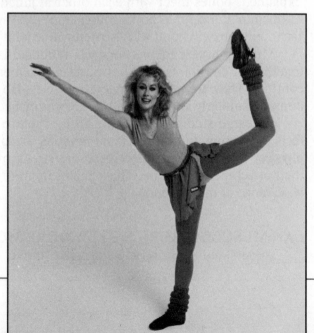

A dancer's coordination is the result of properly developed strength and flexibility.

DO THE BENEFITS OF MUSCLEAEROBICS
OUTWEIGH ADDITIONAL BODY STRESSES?

MuscleAerobics offers many benefits—from increased muscle endurance to improved oxygen capacity and stronger bones.

These benefits are the result of "good" stress. There is "good" stress, and there is "bad" stress. Good stress is activity that pushes you to the next step—greater endurance—leading to better health. Bad stress pushes your body beyond its limits in an effort to get results too fast—never a good idea.

Exercise physiologists have conducted much research dealing with added stress on muscles and bones. They have concluded that *overload training* or increasing your exercise workloads will place good stress on your bones just as it does on your muscles. The large pulling and tugging forces on the bones eventually produce structural changes if the intensity is high enough.

Scientific studies show that this type of overloading increases bone size and density. There is also some evidence that overloading increases bone strength. Other studies have shown that prior physical training can help the healing process in a broken bone.

Initial observations and studies have led to these conclusions, and the benefits of good stress are being tested more and more. What these reports have indicated is that *inactivity* produces a loss of both bone mass and size.

On a related note, it is important to remember that the weight added to your upper body increases the impact to your lower body when running in place. For this reason we recommend a MuscleAerobics program that starts out slow—at a beginner's level. Once your body has adapted to this new challenge, you can feel confident about moving on to more advanced levels.

WHAT IS MUSCLE OVERLOADING IN MUSCLEAEROBICS?

Any time you want to increase the "force capacity" of a muscle, considerable resistance or loads must be applied. These "loads" may be in any form—barbells, dumbbells or your own body weight. Muscles respond to the overload demand itself not to the type of overload. The important thing is that the demand must be of sufficient intensity to cause the body to adapt and change. This is referred to as the *overload principle.*

Overloading with dumbbells is done by increasing the weight, the number of repetitions, or the number of times a particular set of exercises is repeated. Before getting to the specific application of the overload principle, we'll explain how MuscleAerobics evolved from weight training to its present form.

Some History—The overload principle is certainly not new. Milo of Crotona in 500 B.C. "overloaded" by carrying a bull calf on his back every day until the calf reached maturity. Thanks to this "training," he was undefeated as an Olympian wrestler for many years.

Through the ages, man has overloaded by carrying heavy objects or by training with heavy weapons. At the turn of the century, circus strongmen were in vogue. They would achieve tremendous strength by lifting heavy loads for few repetitions.

The overload principle in relation to free weights or dumbbells is best defined as training with heavy weight loads for a few repetitions as opposed to training with light weights for many repetitions.

Absolute strength, in the true sense of the word, is enhanced by overloading with heavy weight for few repetitions in a progressive manner. Heavy weight with few repetitions produces *hypertrophy,* or big muscles. We'll leave that to bodybuilders.

In MuscleAerobics, the best application of overloading involves adding weight *and* increasing repetitions. Any weight you add in MuscleAerobics is for less than you would add with weight training. The highest weight you would ever add is five pounds. We recommend that only for a person who has been on the program at least a couple of years. In fact, we ourselves use two-pound weights, maximum.

Remember, MuscleAerobics increases muscular endurance. Strength training increases muscle mass. The high-repetition training of MuscleAerobics affects the structural and chemical makeup of the muscle fibers, enhancing their ability to use oxygen and produce energy.

Applying the overload principle for several weeks, you'll find what was difficult before becomes easier. This is the body's signal that you are adapting to overload. In other words, you're improving. But to continue to improve in a MuscleAerobics program, you need to increase your intensity continually so you can continue the overload cycle. This results in continuous progression.

We must stress that applying overload in MuscleAerobics is not a weekly progression. It is more a matter of months before your body is truly ready for you to go to the next step. And, the next step may not be with increased weight. It may be running or cycling longer. It may be lifting your feet higher or swinging the weight higher. Generally speaking, overloading is increasing the intensity. And this is what MuscleAerobics is all about. It *is not* a strength or power program.

Above all keep in mind that any overloading program must not be greater than your present conditioning allows. Otherwise, reduced performance and injury will result due to bad stress.

WHY DO I GET GREATER ENDURANCE WITH MUSCLEAEROBICS?

If you don't stress or overload the body somewhat, cardiovascular or muscular endurance won't develop. Animals fully utilize all four limbs in all their activities. While we are not advocating a program in which you run around on all fours, we are recommending that you use your arms and legs to maximum capability.

By adding a weight in your hand, you have created resistance. When you run, the ground and the force of gravity provide a resistance too. In most exercise programs, your arms do not experience this kind of activity. Therefore, they require some type of additional force to impact your cardiovascular system. This additional muscle stress causes positive benefits that eventually make the heart beat more efficiently. It's a total-body involvement. That means a more powerful and well-proportioned body with the ability to endure more.

HOW MUCH WEIGHT IS RIGHT FOR ME?

The first thing to consider is your present endurance and strength. If you are currently doing arm work throughout an aerobic class and find it easy to get through, that's a good sign. You can most generally add one-pound weights to your current routine.

Be sure to move into a MuscleAerobics program carefully. Unweighted arm movements should be easy before you add weight. When you use handweights for the first time, the aerobic arm movements will seem somewhat difficult. If you find that you're doing the arm work in an uncontrolled fashion, slow down or stop using the weights.

Before you continue using the weights, you'll need to develop some additional strength. One recommendation is a daily program of eight to 12 repetitions of slow, controlled pushups. After approximately one month, you should find that this has helped you develop the extra strength needed to begin this exciting program.

WHAT HAPPENS TO MY UPPER BODY?

Working your upper and lower body together will increase cardiovascular fitness to help you achieve maximum endurance levels. You would have to work a lot harder to achieve these levels without the weights. The simultaneous movement of many muscles is an excellent way to train the heart and lungs.

Arms and legs working in combination can perform longer than the legs alone at the same work intensity. MuscleAerobics works to develop balanced strength, endurance and flexibility and gives you a more proportioned physique.

WHAT EXACTLY IS AEROBICS?

Lately, *aerobics* and *fitness* have become almost interchangeable. The two words are closely connected in that aerobics is an integral part of *overall* fitness. But it is also a very specific way of working out.

Overall fitness hinges on the inner workings of your body. You owe it to yourself to have a good understanding of your body and what happens to it when you exercise. With this understanding comes the awareness of MuscleAerobics as a more effective workout than just aerobics alone. We are convinced that this added knowledge will encourage you to learn more.

The following information will help explain aerobic activity and why MuscleAerobics offers great benefits. It is particularly important to understand the major elements that work toward building a stronger heart and lungs, add strength, and create physiological changes that aid in *permanent* weight loss. We will explain why MuscleAerobics is actually aerobics plus much more.

Why You Need Oxygen—There are five basics essential for the survival of man. They are air, food, water, warmth and light. Our relationship with each of these elements is important, but none is as vital as air. Fire cannot burn without oxygen, and neither can we. Oxygen is one reason we survive. Without it we die. That fact alone should give us renewed respect for the air we breathe.

Physiologically, aerobics is a way of making energy by using oxygen. Because oxygen is not stored in the body, we must continually supply it to ourselves every second of the day, whether we are asleep or awake. This is the key to aerobic exercises—proper and efficient use of oxygen.

Aerobics is popular because it improves your level of physical endurance and increases your capacity for performing physical work. The relationship between oxygen consumption and physical activity is of major importance in understanding MuscleAerobics.

HOW DOES ENDURANCE IMPROVE OXYGEN USAGE?

The way to effectively use oxygen is to develop endurance. Endurance is the ability of the muscles to respond to prolonged activity. Three basic elements are necessary to achieve endurance—intensity, duration and frequency.

Training your muscles to respond to prolonged activity requires an exercise program that incorporates steady, *uninterrupted* movement for at least 20 minutes, but ideally 30 minutes, minimally three times a week for cardiovascular benefits. For effective weight loss it should be five times a week.

This type of endurance exercise must also be vigorous enough to cause your oxygen intake to reach a percentage of its maximum level and stay there for at least 15 minutes. This level is determined by your *target heart rate,* discussed in detail later in this chapter.

This system of aerobic exercise was first developed by Dr. Kenneth Cooper. It is now generally supported by the American Heart Association and the President's Council on Physical Fitness as one of the most important methods for acquiring physical fitness.

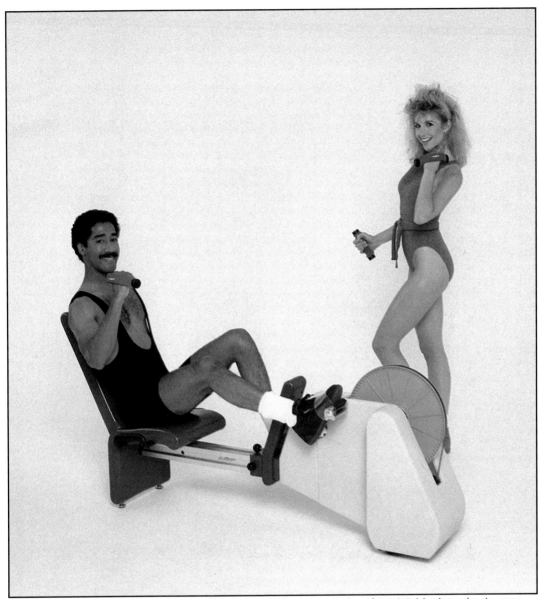

The MuscleAerobics exercises described in chapter 6 offer you a choice of two total-body workouts—one for a stationary bicycle and the other in an aerobics class.

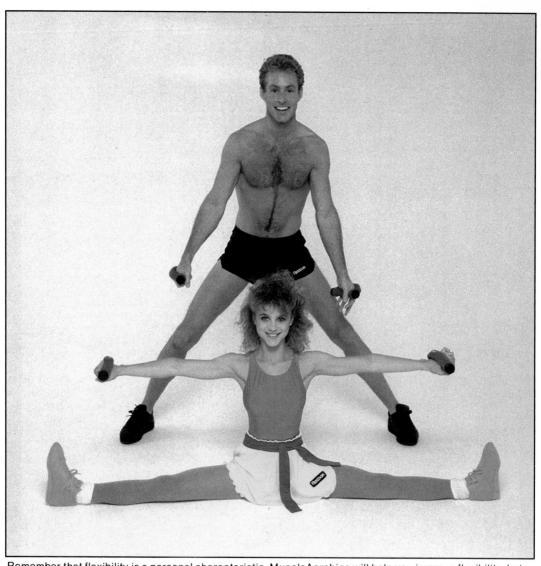

Remember that flexibility is a personal characteristic. MuscleAerobics will help you improve flexibility, but it won't guarantee that you'll ever be able to do splits.

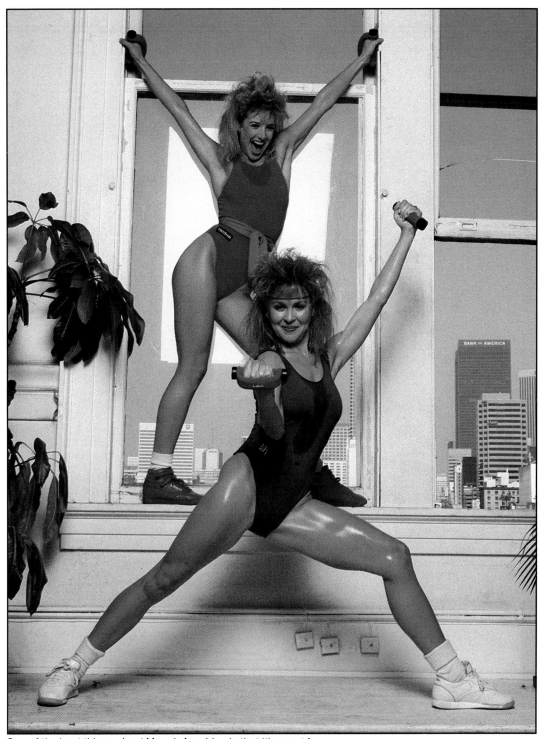

One of the best things about MuscleAerobics is that it's great fun.

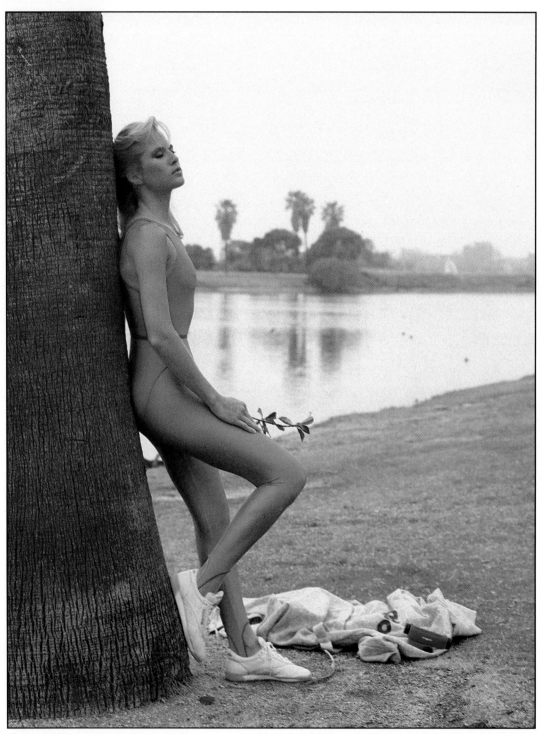

Some quiet relaxation before and after your workout is an important part of the program.

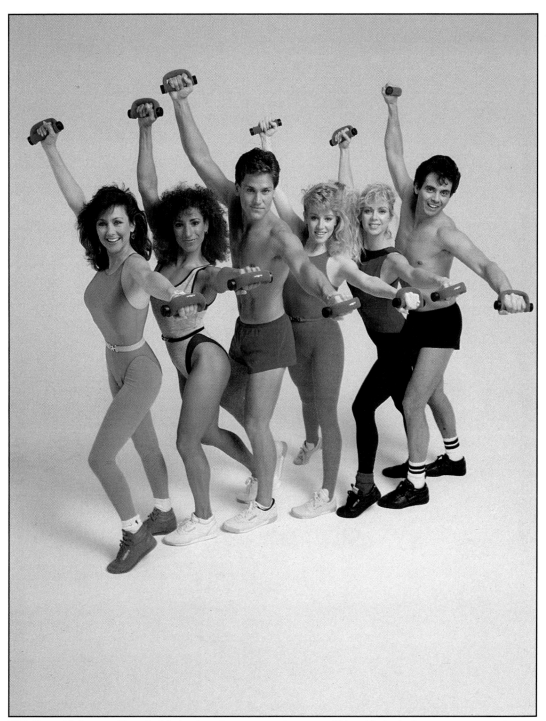

With the guidelines outlined in this book and some experience, you'll be able to design your own exercises, such as the MuscleAerobics Train shown here.

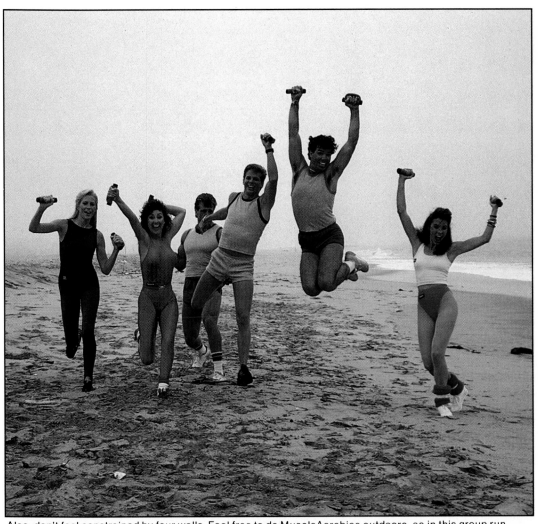

Also, don't feel constrained by four walls. Feel free to do MuscleAerobics outdoors, as in this group run along the beach.

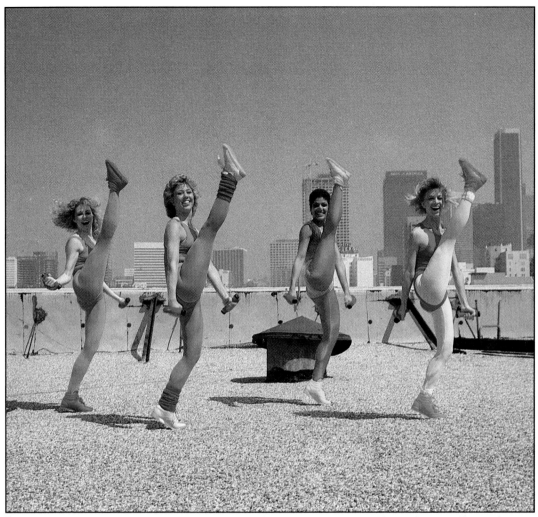

This happy bunch is practicing The Buddy System. As described in the text, MuscleAerobics is more fun and easier to stick with if you consistently work out with a friend or two.

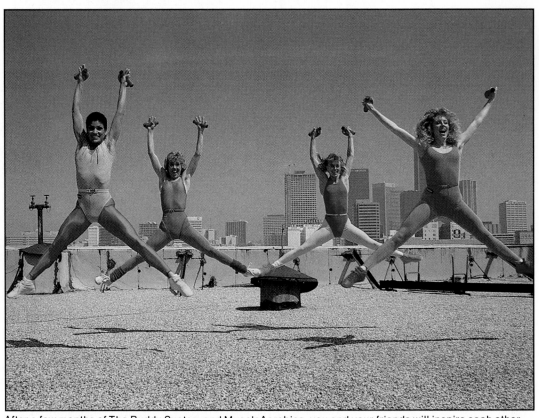

After a few months of The Buddy System and MuscleAerobics, you and your friends will inspire each other to new heights of fitness.

WILL I LOSE WEIGHT DOING MUSCLEAEROBICS?

According to Robert Lawrence, who has developed successful exercise programs, people who exercise five times per week lose weight three times faster than those who exercise only three times per week. And those who exercise only one to two times per week were almost completely ineffectual at losing weight.

Lawrence believes that three times a week will give you a maintenance effect. But five times a week will provide a substantial benefit in weight reduction, if that is your goal.

We agree, and recommend you do a MuscleAerobics program at least five times a week for effective weight loss.

HOW DOES OXYGEN WORK IN MY BODY?

A major role of the cardiovascular system during exercise is the transport of more oxygen to the muscles while exercising. This is achieved both by increasing the volume of blood pumped by the heart and increasing blood flow to active tissues and muscle cells. The following information emphasizes the role of this amazing system in oxygen transport:

For your muscles to contract and lengthen they need oxygen for fuel. As you breathe in oxygen, it is transferred from the lungs to the blood stream and then carried to the heart. The pumping action of your heart causes the oxygen to be transported to the muscles where it is needed.

MuscleAerobics allows the oxygen to be transported to your legs *and* your upper body, because both areas are being worked at the same time and need a supply. This is referred to as the *Oxygen Transport System.*

For the Oxygen Transport System to work effectively, these functions must occur:

1) You must breathe in adequate oxygen from the air.

2) The lungs must take up the oxygen and pass it into the blood.

3) The blood needs to pick up the oxygen delivered by the lungs.

4) The heart must pump blood to all parts of the body.

5) Blood vessels need to be clear so blood can be transported to muscle tissues.

6) Oxygen in the blood is released and picked up by the cells needing it.

7) Cells use the oxygen to produce energy.

8) Cells in turn discard waste products back into the blood.

9) Blood returns these waste products back to the lungs.

10) The lungs will then expel the waste, carbon dioxide. The process begins again.

By using the heart and lungs, this system works to ensure proper delivery of oxygen to the appropriate cells. As this system improves due to the aerobic activity of MuscleAerobics, your *metabolism* changes along with it.

WHAT IS METABOLISM AND HOW CAN MUSCLEAEROBICS IMPROVE IT?

Most medical dictionaries use the word *metabolism* to represent all bodily chemical reactions that require energy. Movement in all living beings requires lots of energy. This energy is provided by various chemical reactions that occur in and around muscle fibers.

Our first source of energy is provided by the food we eat. Once the food is digested, the metabolic processes of the body take over. In other words, metabolism is the result of energy needed for the basic functions in life such as circulation, digestion, respiration, growth, reproduction and so forth.

Energy can't be described in terms of size or shape, it can only be expressed by its ability to produce change. Essentially, the amount of work done is a measure of energy. The extent of the movement and the force of muscular contraction dictates the amount of energy expended. MuscleAerobics places demands on the body that cause greater energy expenditure, thereby increasing your metabolism.

Increasing your metabolism can be compared to the fine-tuning of a car. Just like the engine, MuscleAerobics can tune your body so that it is "humming" along, performing at its peak. It will burn calories with the same productiveness of that perfectly running engine. In short, MuscleAerobics will transform your body from an efficient fat storer to an efficient fat burner.

WHAT IS THE PROCESS OF BURNING CALORIES?

How calories are "burned" is fascinating, but sometimes complex. It's best to define *calorie* first:

Different characteristics of the body are measured with different units. For example, height is usually measured in feet and inches, and weight in pounds. Scientists use calories to measure units of body energy. For example, a 4-oz. baked potato—without butter or sour cream—provides you with approximately 81 units of energy, called calories. Your body needs this energy for fuel.

Obviously, calories are the measurement of energy derived from various types of food that you eat. Two of the most important sources of energy from foods that the body uses are carbohydrates and fats. Of the two, fats are the preferred source of energy that is stored in the body. However, *excess* fat places undue stress on the body in areas such as the arteries and the muscles. Excess fat concerns us most. The prospect of excess fat is what we want to avoid. One of the best ways to get rid of it is through aerobic exercise.

Calories in the form of fats—such as in milk, cream and butter—and carbohydrates—such as in bread, pasta and sweets—are broken down via the digestive system. Fats are broken down into simpler fatty acids. Carbohydrates are broken down and converted into glucose.

Fatty acids and glucose are then transported via the blood to other parts of the body. Fats are stored in fat cells. Glucose is converted into glycogen and then stored in the liver and muscles.

When exercising, muscles "burn" combinations of fat and glucose. As you begin to exercise, your body burns glucose or glycogen for immediate energy. Then fat is released from fat cells. By continuing to exercise aerobically—reaching a certain heart beat and sustaining it for 20 minutes or more—fat becomes released at a faster rate. This way it becomes the preferred source of energy.

In other words, aerobic exercise continually uses fat as its main energy source. MuscleAerobics demands more energy because more work is involved. Therefore, more calories are used. The more calories you use, the more fats you burn, and the more weight you lose. This is one of the greatest benefits of total-body workout.

In summary, MuscleAerobics helps your muscle tissues become more efficient at *oxidizing*—or breaking down—stored body fat because it makes every minute count. A long-term result is an increase in the enzyme responsible for fat oxidation. You become a more efficient fat burner during exercise *and even when you're not exercising.* In addition, your muscles become leaner and you become thinner.

WHY DOES IT TAKE SO LONG TO SEE RESULTS?

Have you ever known people who have been thin all their lives and never exercised, then all of a sudden put on weight? One reason is because these people, who you thought were thin, were actually fat but didn't show it. The reason they finally started to show signs of being overweight is because that fat finally appeared just beneath the surface of the skin.

There are two levels of fat. One is within the muscle, called *intramuscular fat.* The other is beneath the surface of the skin and is called *subcutaneous fat.* Thin people who suddenly appear fat because of improper diet and little exercise were actually accumulating fat within the muscle. New fat finally showed beneath their skin to give the overweight appearance.

Fat loss works almost the same as fat gain, except in reverse. Initially, fat loss occurs within the muscle. Maybe your scale indicates some weight loss, but your body looks the same to you. It is during this time that many people get discouraged and frustrated and quit their program.

As you exercise, your muscles get leaner but you may weigh nearly the same because muscle weighs more than fat. But when you stick with your program, you'll start to see changes because lean muscles mean a thinner, more proportioned body. When the intramuscular fat gets used, your body uses subcutaneous fat. Then you'll see more changes in tone and shape.

WHAT ABOUT PEOPLE WHO DIET AND DON'T EXERCISE?

Aerobic exercise is the *only* way to lose weight and keep it off. And aerobic exercise is the *only* way to lose fat within the muscle. It is almost impossible to remove intramuscular fat by restricting food intake. Dieting alone will not do it.

Dieters who do little else may lose subcutaneous fat, but they still have fat within the muscle. That's why they see the results so soon. And it is why they easily gain back what was lost.

An overweight person who diets and never exercises will always have a weight problem and will always have excess intramuscular fat. The fat cells in the muscles are full. Any extra fat that arrives has to go somewhere—beneath the skin for everyone to see. So, once again, they diet and the vicious cycle continues.

Dieters treat the problem; they don't correct it. The only correction is exercise with an effective program like Muscle Aerobics.

WHAT IS MY TARGET HEART RATE AND HOW DO I USE IT?

During exercise, slow down or stop and place your finger on your pulse, either at the artery in your neck or at your wrist. Count the heart beats for six seconds—starting with 0, 1, 2, etc. Then add a zero. This gives you the number of heart beats per minute.

For example, if at the end of six seconds you counted 13 beats, your heart rate is 130. Your heart rate is your "intensity indicator." You need to be able to read this indicator because each person has a limit as to how much blood the heart can pump and how much oxygen the lungs can consume at a time. Monitoring your heart beats during exercise provides you the gauge for determining your limits. The limit is determined by your target heart rate.

You can figure it out with the following formulas:

$$220 - \text{Your Age} = \text{Maximum Heart Rate (MR)}$$
$$\text{MR} \times (60\% \text{ to } 80\%) = \text{Target Heart Rate (TR)}$$

Your target rate represents your top oxygen-consumption level. An athlete, for example, would work at the 80% level. If you are just starting a fitness program, you should use the 60% figure.

WHAT IF I CAN'T MAINTAIN A STEADY PACE?

Start off by exercising at an even pace without significantly increasing or decreasing your aerobic activity. Determine this by exercising at a level that allows you to talk during the workout. Isn't that part of what exercising is all about—sharing and having fun? Don't work so hard that your muscles can't adapt to the new stress of your workout. No one wants to exercise when it becomes unpleasant and constantly difficult.

A steady pace will allow you to "talk it up" with your fellow exercisers. But don't get carried away to the point where you're really not putting in the required effort. Basically, you want to know that you can at least get a good workout and talk at the same time.

WHAT AEROBIC EXERCISES ARE THERE OTHER THAN RUNNING AND AEROBIC DANCE?

To name a few: jumping rope, bicycling, swimming, cross-country skiing, stationary bicycling, walking. An aerobic exercise is any activity that can be sustained for at least 20 minutes at your target heart rate.

WHY ARE THESE TYPES OF EXERCISES GOOD FOR ME?

The major benefits of aerobic exercises are a stronger and more efficiently operating heart and lungs, more energy, physical flexibility, conditioned muscles, proper use of fats, and effective burning of calories. The increased oxygen flow gained through aerobics re-energizes you, giving you more energy and a "re-awakening" of your senses.

In other words, as the heart pumps more blood with fewer beats, your body systems are in sync, allowing you to take in more oxygen. When everything is operating smoothly, your body can efficiently transport and utilize oxygen with no obstructions.

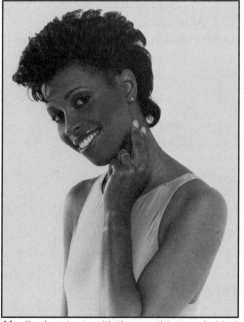 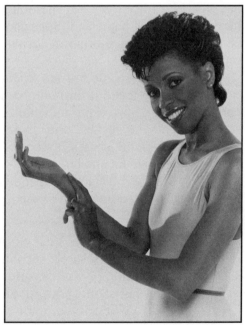

Monitor heart rate with the carotid artery behind your jawbone (left) or at your radial artery on the wrist (right).

The nucleus of this whole system is the heart. Each heart beat is responsible for propelling the oxygenated blood through the proper blood vessels. Aerobic exercise will produce an increased capacity for pumping larger volumes of blood to accommodate the need for extra energy and extra oxygen.

WHAT IS THE ROLE OF GLUCOSE AND GLYCOGEN IF I WANT TO BURN FAT?

When taken into the body, carbohydrates are converted into glucose. Glucose is then transported to the liver via the blood. In the liver it is turned into glycogen.

The body burns combinations of fats and glucose for fuel. Glucose burning for energy takes place in two stages during exercise. The first stage is the *anaerobic* phase, where very little oxygen is needed. The second stage, the aerobic phase, needs lots of oxygen. Glucose acts as fuel when working anaerobically.

WHAT IS ANAEROBICS?

Anaerobic means *without oxygen.* Here's an example when it comes into play: Suppose you are working out or running so fast that you can hardly catch your breath. More than likely, you're exceeding your target heart rate. Being able to do the activity for a short time indicates that you were using your anaerobic capacity rather than your aerobic capacity. In other words, you're working harder than your heart and lungs can handle. As a result, the total amount of energy that can be produced during this phase is limited by your anaerobic capacity.

Glycogen has to be burned in two stages. By substantially exceeding your training rate, glycogen is burned only in the first stage—the anaerobic one. Not enough oxygen has been metabolized to continue the process through the second stage—the aerobic one. In this case, you can say that during the first stage all fat-burning ceases. Essentially you use glycogen as your main energy source rather than fat and oxygen.

To work aerobically, you need oxygen and fats as fuel. To work anaerobically, you don't need oxygen, just glucose as your fuel.

IS MUSCLEAEROBICS EVER ANAEROBIC?

Yes, even though MuscleAerobics is mostly an aerobic activity. With any type of aerobic activity, you can move out of the aerobic phase and into the anaerobics phase by significantly increasing intensity.

Here's why: When you are not exercising, the amount of energy you need for everyday activities is so small that you don't need much oxygen. But when you exercise, your breathing increases and your body needs more oxygen.

After you have warmed up and proceed to more accelerated movements, such as a quick jog, your body needs energy right away.

Physiologically, this means that the rate of oxygen transport has to catch up with the rate of your jogging. Luckily, your body is prepared to handle it. It maintains an emergency backup system—the spark to ignite your body to keep it going. This needed supply of energy comes from stored glycogen.

This is not unlike your car when you start it. When you put the key in the ignition and turn it, the first thing that is activated is the battery. Once the engine is running, it relies on the generator and gasoline to keep it going.

Believe it or not, your body reacts similarly. During the beginning stages of your workout, you are working anaerobically. Your body's battery power, glycogen, gets you going. As you continue the intensity of your exercise routine, your body relies on its generator, the oxygen transport system, to take over. When this happens, you have begun to work aerobically.

As mentioned, aerobic activities have to be steady and uninterrupted to give the greatest benefits. It is possible after reaching this aerobic stage to once again move into an anaerobic phase.

Here's how: All you have to do is introduce more vigorous activity. This will cause you to exceed your target heart rate. For example, professional long-distance runners train in the following way to develop speed. They may run for approximately 5 to 10 miles, sprint for one mile, run for an additional five miles, and sprint again.

Five miles of running for most people is typically more than 30 minutes of aerobic activity. Keep in mind that this type of training is geared to improving racing times. The average person is not concerned with racing times in an aerobic class or on a stationary bicycle.

So when you're dealing with *only* 30 minutes of aerobic activity, you want to make every minute count. In other words, you want to avoid a program involving a continual change from high-intensity to low-intensity action. That causes you to consistently move from an aerobic to an anaerobic phase. This results in an improper use of fats.

In a MuscleAerobics program, it's better to start off with a slow jog while pumping your arms in front of you. Slowly increase the intensity, eventually lifting your knees up higher and pumping your arms over your head and maintaining the intensity for at least 20 minutes. To end, go back to the slow jog again.

This way, you continue using fats as your major fuel source, saving glycogen for "emergencies."

On a related note, pushing yourself far beyond your training rate will create a painful buildup of *lactic acid* in the muscles.

WHAT IS LACTIC ACID?

When the intensity of the exercise is so great that not enough oxygen can be delivered to muscles, an *oxygen debt* develops. This is caused by either a lag in the circulatory transport of oxygen to the working muscles, a lag in the metabolic reactions of the cells and tissues, or both.

Whatever the reason, the result is an oxygen-consumption imbalance. A lag occurs between the time your body delivers oxygen and the actual consumption of it. This "phase lag" is the *oxygen debt.* During the phase lag, a chemical reaction within the muscle occurs, producing lactic acid.

For example, have you ever experienced difficulty breathing when you were exercising, but you didn't want to stop? After a while, you might have found that you had no choice but to slow down or stop because of pain in your muscles. Unless you injured yourself, this pain was probably due to lactic acid buildup. You could say that lactic acid is one way for your body to tell you to stop or slow down.

To reduce lactic acid buildup, you need to slow down, allowing the oxygen to flow back into the painful muscle. The oxygen pays the oxygen debt, permitting you to catch your breath and continue the routine.

This same principle can apply to weightlifting. Powerlifters, bodybuilders and weightlifters can lift only so much weight so many times. Have you every tried to lift a heavy weight and were only able to lift it a few times, if that? If someone wanted you to lift it one more time, you probably couldn't . It was as if your arms turned to rubber. But if you paused for a few minutes and tried to lift the weight again, you may have discovered that you were able to lift it a few times again.

Your lack of ability was most likely due to lactic acid buildup. "Curing" lactic acid buildup means allowing oxygen to flow back into your muscles to "rejuvenate" muscle cells so they can keep working.

ARE THERE BENEFITS FROM EXERCISING ANAEROBICALLY?

Yes. Most anaerobic-type exercises assist in acquiring strength, increasing muscle tone and in developing speed. Unfortunately, anaerobic workouts cannot be continued long enough to burn fat.

For example, weightlifters can lift only so many repetitions of heavy weight at a time. Within minutes they have to stop and rest because they have exhausted the muscle. Sprinters can not possibly sustain for 15 minutes the fast speeds at which they run a 50-yard dash.

The weightlifter and the sprinter are working harder than their heart can pump blood and their lungs can consume oxygen. They are using their anaerobic capacity, which doesn't require large amounts of oxygen or fats for fuel.

IS RACQUETBALL AN AEROBIC SPORT?

Many sports and activities can be vigorous without being aerobic. According to guidelines by the American College of Sports Medicine (ACSM), cardiovascular fitness is related to the intensity, duration and frequency of training. The ACSM suggests the following for anaerobic activities:

1) Frequency should be three to five times per week.

2) Intensity should be within 60% to 90% of the maximum heart rate, or 50% to 85% of the maximum oxygen intake.

3) Duration should be 15 to 60 minutes of continuous activity.

Generally, racquetball is not considered an aerobic activity because most players don't fulfill the three criteria mentioned. But a recent study conducted by members of the Department of Medicine at the University of Arkansas for Medical Sciences monitored the heart rates of 15 racquetball players during a singles competition. They concluded that during a one-hour singles match, subjects attained "an average of 83% of the maximum heart rate and played above 60% of the maximum heart rate for 56 continuous minutes." "However," the study continued, "the conclusion cannot be drawn from the present study or one performed with professionals that racquetball produces a good cardiovascular-fitness level in an individual."

The study was conducted with amateur racquetball players and professional racquetball players. Different results were obtained, indicating that the more proficient you are at the game, the less moving around you do. Therefore you are creating stop and go movements, constituting anaerobic activity.

Some other typical anaerobic activities include: tennis, football, baseball and volleyball. All involve vigorous play with stop and go movements. Such sports make the cardiovascular system work hard, but only in short bursts. Aerobic training requires steady, continuous work.

HOW CAN MUSCLEAEROBICS BE AEROBIC
IF WEIGHTLIFTING IS ANAEROBIC?

As long as you can sustain an activity for at least 20 minutes with or without weights, you are working aerobically. MuscleAerobics uses weights you can lift with ease, allowing you to raise, lower and swing your arms. Typically, weights heavier than five pounds would be difficult to maneuver when you are running in an aerobics class or riding on a stationary bicycle.

A MUSCLEAEROBICS SUMMARY

We've given you some insight into two very important body systems that are involved during exercise—your muscular and cardiovascular systems.

No machine, even in these days of advanced technology, is as important as your body. Just like a good mechanic who has to know his machinery, we should know our bodies before we start tinkering with them. The whole concept of our marvelous body machine and the benefits gained from productive use of it is the essence of MuscleAerobics.

We've mentioned that to achieve overall fitness, your workout must incorporate endurance, flexibility, toning and strengthening exercises. A MuscleAerobics program offers all of them. It truly is a complete program.

Weight Control—Being overweight or obese are problems for a large segment of our population. MuscleAerobics can contribute to weight control in several ways. Perhaps the most obvious is by increasing the body's energy needs. MuscleAerobics increases your expenditure of calories. Needless to say, the more calories you burn, the more weight you lose—if you don't increase food intake.

Of course, if you are considerably overweight, MuscleAerobics should be combined with some form of reduced calorie intake to produce significant weight loss.

A less obvious effect of MuscleAerobics is a better body shape. Overweight persons who adopt a MuscleAerobics program often initially experience a loss of inches more than weight loss. Studies indicate that regular aerobic exercise alone contributes to weight control by increasing your metabolism rate. Because MuscleAerobics uses more energy than most regular exercise, you are increasing your caloric expenditure not only during the program but also following the program.

Stronger Heart and Lungs—Dr. Kenneth Cooper provided evidence indicating that aerobic-type exercise affects cardiovascular and respiratory function by increasing the size of existing blood vessels and making them more elastic. This reduces resistance to blood flow and results in lower blood pressure.

MuscleAerobics will significantly improve your cardiovascular system because it is an aerobic-plus exercise program. Therefore, it will increase your heart size and strength, enabling your heart to pump more blood with each stroke—during exercise and at rest.

All this results in a lowered *resting heart rate*. Your heart will rest more between contractions. In other words, by strengthening the heart, you've increased its efficiency as a pump. A heart that beats more slowly and less frequently requires less oxygen for its own work.

Better Muscular Endurance—By improving muscular endurance throughout your body, you will be able to continue any activity or sport for longer periods of time without tiring. MuscleAerobics doesn't mean that you achieve muscular endurance only in your legs. The program is complete because it includes the upper body too.

In addition, the development of greater muscular endurance reduces the risk of muscle tears and other injuries because injury primarily occurs in overly fatigued muscles. Once you've improved your muscular endurance, you've significantly reduced your chances of being injured during exercise.

Stronger Bones—In a recently reported study conducted in England with more than 100 women with broken hips, researchers concluded that the greatest single factor setting the stage for fracture was not a deficiency of calcium, vitamin D or estrogen. Rather, this factor was a deficiency of daily physical activity. Patients with fractures were similar to other patients in every respect, except in regard to their fitness level.

Inactivity leads to thin and vulnerable bones, especially in women. As you grow older, there's a tendency for your bones to lose calcium and become weak and brittle. As a result, fractures and breaks can become a real threat. This is possible even if you sustain a light fall by simply stepping off a sidewalk curb.

Studies continue to show that bone strength is related to aerobic exercise. Dr. Kenneth Cooper reported examples of serious tennis players who tend to have larger and stronger bones in their playing arm than in their other arm. Cooper also mentioned that weightlifters have thicker arm bones than runners. So naturally the stronger and thicker your bones, the less prone to fractures you'll become as you get older.

Improved Body Awareness—Fitness starts with a *balanced* and *centered* body. *Balanced* means that the weight of your body is distributed evenly. *Centered* means that your body position is concentrated and movements are initiated from the physical center of your body. By combining mind, body, motion and technique through MuscleAerobics, you'll gain a mastery over the elements of balance and coordination.

Flexibility plays a significant role in body awareness. Because most day-to-day forms of physical activity do not require muscles to go through their full range of motion, people who don't actively exercise their muscles are less flexible than those who do.

Sharper Mental Awareness—Basically, it is the mind that controls our workouts. It dictates the amount and length of our exercise programs. It is the mind that gets you through the last situp or helps you make that last repetition. Even so, it wasn't until recent years that researchers began to concentrate on the mind's role relative to the body. Today, research is causing us to think in terms of a healthy brain as part of a healthy body. And a healthy body provides a healthier mental and emotional life.

Studies have shown that exercise releases and helps produce chemicals in the brain that enhance intellectual awareness. We're sure that with a daily MuscleAerobics program, you will have more energy and good feelings than you have right now. When fatigued, you cannot perform to your potential. The more healthy and energetic you become, the more you will accomplish.

Positive Self-Image—What we see in the current fitness boom is society participating in a grand experiment. We hope that as more people become fit, they will all start feeling better about themselves. It's only natural, especially when we notice positive changes in our physical shape and fitness.

It becomes obvious that much of our emotional well-being is dependent upon our self-image. When we feel good about ourselves, it penetrates our barrier of self-consciousness, allowing our real selves freedom to shine through.

A survey conducted by *Psychology Today* magazine found that "many Americans who feel powerless to effect changes in their private lives find that physical health is their last bastion of personal control—something that they themselves can influence." The main thing we'd like to emphasize is that, while exercise is not the final answer to an improved self-image, our physical well-being plays a significant role in determining how we feel about ourselves.

Basic Training—MuscleAerobics is basic training. The total-workout concept helps prepare the entire body for day-to-day activities as well as for specific sports. To that end, the exercises in chapter 6 are designed to emulate specific sports activities. You will mimic movements with applied upper-body resistance. This trains you for actual performance of similar moves.

For example, by pumping light handweights in an up and down fashion above your head during MuscleAerobics, you are also training for activity on the volleyball court.

A MuscleAerobics program helps you to be a prepared weekend athlete, whether your sport is golf, tennis or boxing. A conscientious MuscleAerobics training program offers the most vital components of a total exercise program—aerobic activity, muscular endurance and training for the whole body.

The benefits derived from such a total exercise program far exceed any other regime we've ever come across. And we're not alone! Anyone we've introduced to MuscleAerobics soon became hooked. One reason is that you feel the results right away. It's a better workout in a shorter period of time.

The brief case studies in chapter 8 will give you an opportunity to review the progress of first-time MuscleAerobics participants. But now it's time to start training.

CHAPTER FOUR

Starting Out

Just about everyone is getting involved in fitness today. The proof lies in crowded health clubs and streets busy with joggers and bicyclists. A Sunday stroll in many public parks and beaches will surround you with throngs of bicyclists, roller skaters and joggers. It's obvious that most people want to get fit *and have fun* at the same time. In a sense that's the best reason we know for the ultimate workout—producing the most fun and benefits.

It also seems that every week a new exercise book or plan appears. Take a quick glance through the health section of your local bookstore and you'll discover at least two or three shelves of such books. Also, notice what most of the books have in common—aerobic exercise!

Physiologists have proved it time and again. You can't ignore it anymore: Aerobic exercise is necessary for weight loss, weight maintenance and an all-around healthy life. As discussed in chapter 3, aerobic exercise is the foundation of MuscleAerobics.

Whether you are most interested in weight loss or body shaping, remember that weight gain or bad tone doesn't happen overnight. Obviously, correcting these problems won't happen overnight either. Even so, MuscleAerobics will work for you—and also those of you who just want to have a total-body fitness program that is fun and healthy.

START GRADUALLY

Whether you're in shape or out of shape, you should adjust to MuscleAerobics gradually. If you are a newcomer to fitness, you'll be embarking on a new lifestyle. MuscleAerobics allows you to start slowly and carefully increase your fitness level.

For those of you already in shape, you'll discover how quickly your body will adapt to MuscleAerobics workouts. Handling weights while running in place in an aerobics class or moving your arms on a stationary bicycle is a new challenge, but an exciting one. You, too, should start out slowly and build up gradually.

EFFICIENT RESULTS

Your next question probably is, "When do I see the results?" In our experience, people doing MuscleAerobics experience results associated with more oxygenated blood in three days.

We can safely say that within three months you'll really *feel* the difference all over. In six months you'll *see* the difference. In one year, you will have *made* the difference. Don't put the book down just because a year sounds too long. Don't worry. Just *feeling* the difference will give you a useful, long-term attitude about exercise. Many body types respond much sooner, and yours just might be one. But if you're at least 25 pounds overweight or significantly out of shape, the 3-, 6- and 12-month timetable appears more realistic.

HOW TO START

Previous chapters dealt with basics and some physiology of exercise, especially MuscleAerobics. You've learned about the many benefits offered through MuscleAerobics, and now you're ready to begin the program.

We'll start you slowly, so you get a good awareness of your physical condition. You'll be happier if you start with a program suited for your fitness level. This will help decrease the chance of frustration and discouragement that easily arise as you begin.

STEP 1: COMPONENTS OF FITNESS

To determine fitness level, it is helpful to know the actual *components of fitness.* These are the elements that comprise a healthy person. Researchers and educators use a statistical technique to decide which components are common to all sports or fitness programs. Rather than dealing with this scientific approach, we've focused on three important elements—*strength, flexibility* and *endurance.* These three areas provide a good foundation for a well-rounded fitness program.

Strength—This is merely a measure of how strong you are. Technically, strength deals with the force capacity of muscle—in other words, not how big your muscle is, but how strong.

Strength is the functional component. It is involved in everything we do. It is what keeps our body parts in place. Strength is necessary not only for lifting,

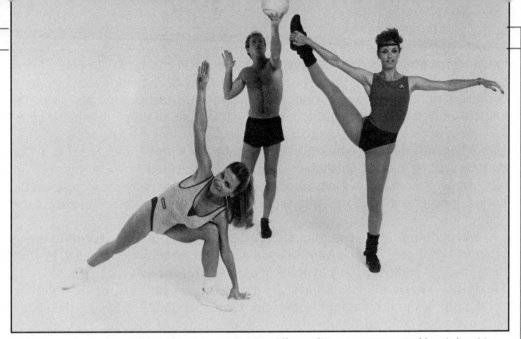

Activities such as yoga, volleyball and dance develop different fitness components. MuscleAerobics provides all three—strength, flexibility and endurance.

but also for simple tasks such as standing up and sitting down. Whether you are walking to the store or running a marathon, strength is required.

An important thing to remember is that strong muscles will work for you and never against you. "But how much strength is enough?" you ask. One expert says that to properly answer that question, you must determine what you use your strength for and why you want more—if you do. He also points out that you can't develop muscle strength until you have some muscle bulk to work with.

MuscleAerobics provides you the training to acquire muscle bulk that will help you excel in a sport. MuscleAerobics will not make you look like a weightlifter, but it will give you enough muscular endurance for just about any other activity.

There are different aspects of strength—*power, force* and *static strength.* Power is seen in quick movements when you move your body weight either upward or forward. For example, you exhibit power when you jump, as did gold-medal hurdler Edwin Moses in the 1984 Summer Olympics. Strength as an explosive force is also found in activities using force on an external object, such as shot or discus.

Static strength is used by applying strength to an external object that doesn't move. This is also called an *isometric contraction*—the testing of the muscle's *maximum force capacity.*

To understand this, play Superman for a second. Stand in a doorway and extend your arms out. Push against the frame and try to break it open. This is isometric contraction of your arm muscles. The measurement is static strength because you're not moving anything, but you are using muscular strength. Some women will remember the isometric contraction of pressing palms together at shoulder level to try to increase bust size.

When only body weight is lifted repeatedly but with significant difficulty for each repetition, as in pushups, strength is measured by the number of repetitions. You may not have associated continuous movement with strength, but it is a necessary and important aspect in strength development and muscular endurance.

Strength and muscle endurance can be increased in a variety of exercise programs. But only MuscleAerobics will give you muscular endurance in your upper body in addition to the benefits of aerobic exercise.

Flexibility—In simple terms, *flexibility* means lack of stiffness, or the ability to bend easily without breaking. In exercise terms, flexibility is having the ability to move your body and limbs through a wide range of motion. This involves stretching muscles and tissues around joints.

Flexibility exercises have become an essential element in conditioning. An effective stretching program involves all major muscles and joints to improve flexibility. Stretching also increases blood flow. It elongates the muscles being stretched and relieves tension in those muscles. Basically, stretching can aid athletic performance, lower the chance of injury, and simply feel good. But you must do it right. One writer calls this *training, not straining.*

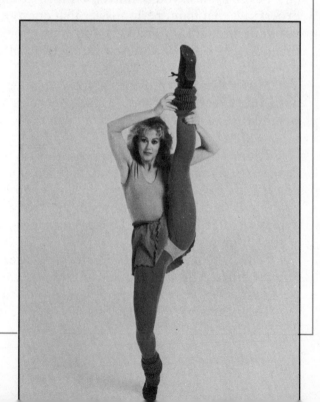

Flexibility improves through training, not straining.

Not everybody can do the same stretching exercises. Most exercise experts consider flexibility an *individual* and *variable* characteristic. No two people have the same degree of flexibility. A stretch that is good for you may not help another person at all.

Stretching exercises help enhance performance and reduce injuries by increasing joint flexibility. Many athletes make the mistake of working only the areas they think contribute to their particular sport. For example, football players are known to be extremely inflexible and have made themselves susceptible to injuries. Realizing this coaches have incorporated strength, conditioning and flexibility programs into practices. Injuries have decreased.

There are two basic kinds of flexibility stretches— *ballistic* and *static.* Ballistic stretching involves a substantial amount of movement, so it has bobbing or jerking motions. You've probably seen this type of stretching in an aerobics class, where the exercise instructor may bounce while in a stretched position.

Another ballistic type of flexibility is called *dynamic flexibility.* It requires your legs or arms to move rapidly throughout a large range of movement, such as in swimming. Dynamic flexibility is difficult to assess for many technical reasons, but be assured that great athletes have it.

Static stretching requires minimal movement. Typically, you place your body in a particular stretch position and then slowly and gradually move through a range of motion. You hold the position for a moment before relaxing.

For example, when doing any type of stretching, your range of motion depends on the pliability of tissues and muscles surrounding specific joints. Sit down with your legs extended in front of you. "Walk" your hands down your legs trying to reach your ankles. When you've reached the farthest point, slowly bend forward trying to touch your chest to your knees. When you can't bend down any farther, hold the position for approximately 20 seconds before relaxing and returning to the starting position.

Your range of motion can be from practically straight up to hands on knees, or all the way down with chin on knees.

Although both stretching techniques may improve flexibility, exercise physiologists agree that static stretching causes fewer injuries. Bouncing during stretching can cause muscle soreness and small tears. When you bounce during a stretch, you trigger a reflex action causing the muscle to contract instead of relax. This type of movement increases your chances of tissue injury.

Static stretching reacts just the opposite. By slowly and gradually placing your body into a position, you let the muscle relax. It is now protected from tearing.

Another benefit of flexibility is the fact that it has been proven to reduce the common aches and pains we develop as we age. Flexibility usually decreases as we get older. Most experts believe that a well-rounded program of stretching will counteract this decline.

Endurance—What do the following activities have in common? Carrying groceries from the car to the kitchen, running to catch the bus, pushing a child in a stroller, and walking up and down stairs all day while housecleaning. The answer is endurance.

To perform any of these everyday activities, you need both muscular and cardiovascular endurance. This is the ability to sustain repeated muscular effort and maintain the intensity. In other words, it refers to the number of repetitions a muscle can perform before exhaustion. To make these everyday activities as effortless as possible, endurance training should be a part of your fitness regime.

There are basically two types of endurance—muscular and cardiovascular endurance. You may argue that the heart is a muscle too, so why the different classifications? As we said, the heart is an involuntary muscle. It requires a certain type of training to get stronger. That's what cardiovascular, or aerobic, exercise is for. Cardiovascular endurance is developed by the continuous, rhythmic movement of aerobic exercise, such as running, swimming, bicycling, jumping rope or cross-country skiing.

Muscular endurance deals specifically with muscle groups. A runner and bicyclist will develop muscular endurance in the legs. Baseball players develop muscular endurance in their arms and shoulders. Muscular endurance can also be developed by various training programs designed to increase strength.

In MuscleAerobics, muscular and cardiovascular endurance are closely interrelated. In MuscleAerobics, you develop cardiovascular endurance during the running portion of the class. You improve muscular endurance through use of handweights and arm movements.

As discussed in chapter 3, you need to consider duration, intensity and frequency when exercising to improve endurance. Benefits result from sustained exercise, as determined by your heart rate and the number of times per week you do it. Don't be misled by sports or activities that make you sweat and breathe hard. Endurance is developed only by sustained and continuous movement.

With all these examples, endurance may be needed to *perform* the exercise, but the exercises in themselves *do not provide* endurance. You need all three elements—duration, intensity and frequency—to develop endurance.

STEP 2: ARE YOU READY PHYSICALLY?

How do you measure your fitness level? First of all, you must truthfully evaluate your present physical capabilities. An important thing to remember when beginning any fitness program is to be realistic. If you are a beginner, don't be ashamed to admit it and start at the beginning. Being honest with yourself will give you the positive results you're looking for. When you read the fitness-level qualifications, keep the following things in mind:

• When was the last time you participated in any type of exercise on a regular basis?

• Were they aerobic-type exercises or sports activities?

• Do you consider yourself an active person?

• What is your age?

• What is your medical history?

• Are you overweight?

• How long have you been overweight?

• If you've been involved in an exercise program before, was your program 30 minutes long, or longer?

If it has been a year or more since you've exercised, you should automatically place yourself in a beginning category. If you are considerably overweight or if you have been inactive for a long time, consult your physician for any customized changes to the beginning MuscleAerobics program.

If you've done only weightlifting or anaerobic exercises with no endurance training, you might have difficulty meeting the stamina requirements.

Have a complete physical before engaging in any strenuous exercise program if you are over 35 and/or have any medical problems. Remember, be honest with yourself. Participating in a 30-minute exercise program three times a week for a year does not necessarily qualify you to enter an advanced level.

The chart on the next two pages provides minimum requirements for determining strength, flexibility and endurance. Your test results will help give you a better idea of your present fitness level. But before beginning the test, please follow these exercise guidelines:

1) Begin toe-touches by curving your head forward, rounding your back, while you let your head weight pull you down. Roll back up with your knees relaxed. Don't bounce up and down.

2) Stand up straight with your back pressed against a wall and feet shoulder-width apart. Relax your knees. Without leaning forward, move your right hand down the right side of your leg as far as you can reach. Repeat with the other side. This set constitutes one count.

3) The purpose of a trunk flexion is to determine the flexibility of the muscles of your back and hamstrings, the back-thigh muscles. Sit on the floor with your legs fully extended and feet flexed. Toes should point upward. Without rounding your back, try to reach for your toes. You should not bounce to get lower or reach farther.

4) Most physical-fitness tests include a distance run to measure endurance. For example, Dr. Kenneth Cooper uses the 12-minute endurance test. We use *chair stepping* and a *walk/run* instead. Chair stepping is done with a sturdy bench, chair or step approximately 15 to 17 inches high. Step up and down every five

Determining Your Fitness Level

FLEXIBILITY

	Toe Touches	Side Stretches	Trunk Flexion
ADVANCED	15 reaches to toes.	15 per side, reaching past knee.	Touch toes and hold for 20 seconds.
INTERMEDIATE	10 reaches to ankles.	10 per side, reaching to knee.	Touch ankles and hold for 20 seconds.
BEGINNING	5 reaches to lower calves.	Reaching maximum stretch, holding for 20 seconds on either side.	Reach for knees and hold for 20 seconds.

ENDURANCE

	Brisk Walking or	Jogging/ Running or	Chair Stepping
ADVANCED	2 miles in less than 25 minutes.	2 miles in less than 16 minutes.	95—134 beats.
INTERMEDIATE	1-1/2 miles in less than 25 minutes.	1-1/2 miles in less than 16 minutes.	135—184 beats.
BEGINNING	1 mile in less than 25 minutes.	Run/walk 2 miles in 25 minutes.	185—229 beats.

Determining Your Fitness Level (cont.)

STRENGTH

	Situps	Modified Pushups
ADVANCED	30 in less than 60 seconds.	15
INTERMEDIATE	20 in less than 60 seconds.	10
BEGINNING	5 in less than 60 seconds.	5

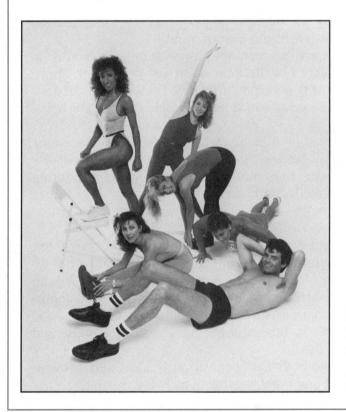

These are the exercises you should do for self-evaluation. If the majority of your results falls into one category, such as *intermediate,* then that's your fitness level. If in doubt about your level, start as a beginner.

seconds for one minute. When you stop, take your pulse immediately for two minutes. Count the *total number* of beats.

5) Do situps with knees bent and feet flat on the floor. Curl your head forward with your arms crossed in front of your chest. A full situp begins when you've curled your shoulders and your upper back is off the floor.

6) In modified pushups, knees are bent and buttocks tucked under. For a complete pushup, the chest is approximately one inch from the floor before pushing off.

STEP 3: MIND OVER MUSCLE

The saying goes that in every fat man or woman, there is a fit person struggling to get out. If this is so, then every fit person must have images of himself or herself with more muscles and strength.

The athlete in each of us is more than an abstract ideal. It is a living presence that can change the way we feel and live. Searching for your inner athlete has led you to MuscleAerobics and thus to the fitness levels you desire.

But no exercise program can be successful without the ancient concept of unified body and mind. Our studies have shown us time and again that proper mental focus is the only way to achieve physical accomplishment and commitment. Therefore, a fit lifestyle begins in your mind.

Today sports psychologists are concerned not only with improving athletic performance but with the athlete's welfare in sport as well. With more scientists, doctors, families and the general public involved in sports, athletic accomplishments are growing every year. World and Olympic records are being surpassed time and again.

As a result, pressures increase on athletes, who are training at a younger age and more intensively than ever before. More and more people are recognizing that athletes' thought processes and emotions immediately before, during and after competition can greatly influence their present and future achievements. In other words, the psychological aspect may work *for or against* the athlete.

As "everyday athletes," we are not subjected to the same pressures, but we're not immune to psychological pressures either. The mind's influence on sports and exercise is much more important than most people realize. We can be plagued with the risks of high-blood pressure, heart attacks and even anorexia nervosa! What about the social pressures of always having to look good? The right psychological approach to fitness is having a positive attitude and determination to be the best you can be.

The combination of mind and body has been variously addressed throughout history. We stress that mind and body are functionally interrelated. To pay attention to one without the other ignores the whole person. A healthy brain is part of a healthy body.

Are You Ready Mentally?—Once you've completed the fitness test, you know the category you're in. We hope that you are physically ready to begin a MuscleAerobics program. But you may still have questions crossing your mind. For example, are you unsure how you feel about starting this program? You may be trying to figure out how serious you are. Along with that, you may be questioning your follow-through.

All of these concerns have to do with mental preparedness. You should be ready to start and stay on your program. But let's face it: Getting started may not be easy. In fact, starting requires as much mental effort as physical—especially when your muscles start to ache, or when you worry about getting injured.

After starting a program, you may get impatient or have mixed feelings. At one point you may be excited; at another time you may be confused by unfamiliar sensations.

STEP 4: COMMITMENT

This is a necessary mental process in a fit lifestyle. As in any battle, especially the "battle of the bulge," specific plans and strategies are necessary to win. We have some suggestions to help you plan emotionally for this mental adventure. We'll give you ways to enjoy it, the dynamics to cope with it and a program to stick with it.

Set Realistic Goals—Discouragement is the first enemy of any exercise program. There is a way to overcome this problem, however, and that is to prepare for it. Once you realize it's going to happen, you can build the fortress to keep it away. One of the most important weapons against discouragement is to begin your program by setting realistic goals. No step is too small if it gets you to the next one.

We've already mentioned that you should start on a beginning MuscleAerobics program only after you have determined that your fitness level is appropriate to proceed. Even if you have been involved in an ongoing fitness program, the added demands of MuscleAerobics can make you feel like a beginner. To meet this challenge you have to take the first step in setting realistic goals, and that is to *oversimplify*.

Your first achievement may be as simple as buying a pair of one-pound handweights. The second can be taking them to an aerobics class. And the third might be to use them for five minutes.

Being realistic also means knowing yourself. If you buy a pair of handweights but feel out of place in your aerobics class, then make it your goal to start a program at home. Test it out first. You might also decide to encourage someone else in class to try out the program with you.

Don't expect to move to an advanced program immediately. The erroneous thinking in this case is that more is better—that more yields faster results.

Write Them Down—Realistic goals involve documentation and review. When setting personal goals, we usually underestimate the amount of time required for a task. Generally, we're off the mark by as much as 50%. So keep in mind that whatever you want to accomplish may take you much longer than you anticipated or hoped. Start by actually writing down your long-range goals.

With the records you can put your program into proper perspective. Then write down your two-month goals, three-month goals and eight-month goals. Use ink! Long-range goals may include losing five pounds, running a 5000-meter race in 25 minutes, finishing a 20-minute MuscleAerobics workout without stopping, or maybe just fitting into a tight pair of old jeans and actually being able to close the top button.

In longer terms, you may want to consider more general goals, such as a better all-around physique, increased endurance, a weight loss of 10 pounds or just continuing a fit lifestyle. These larger goals can then be broken down to more manageable short-term goals. You decide what's important to you and find an appropriate time slot for that goal.

But remember to set your goals carefully. It takes time for the body to adapt to this new type of activity, especially if you've been relatively inactive. Don't let anyone intimidate you into moving faster than you are able to. Remember the 3-, 6-, and 12-month timeline? Your goal is to get in shape and stay in shape. You want it to last a lifetime, not just one summer.

And don't forget: Without a goal, you'll never know when you'll get there. First establish where "there" is—it's your personal goal and no one else's.

Have Fun—Whatever exercise program you choose, make it fun. Even though MuscleAerobics is primarily designed to be performed in a health-club environment, don't feel locked into that setting. Start off where you'll feel most comfortable. After starting out, concentrate on the small pleasures along the way.

It is important to focus on the feeling you get when you meet your first goal. You've worked hard and you've seen the results and that is a very rewarding feeling. As you progress in your fitness regime, you'll feel more confident. You'll be experiencing the sensation of being in better control of your body—you're dictating its future. Rather than going from day to day saying, "I *hope* my heart will stay healthy, my bones strong, my skin vibrant," you *guarantee* it through MuscleAerobics.

Stick to It—There will be times when the burden of exercising can be so heavy that it seems unbearable. To counteract this, we've developed a MuscleAerobics "Buddy System." Share your goals with a partner who also wants to get in shape and has made a commitment just like you. Your buddy's duty is to help motivate you to not miss workouts. You gain moral support through the tough times, and then you do the same for your partner.

Because you've both made the same commitment you have something in common. And because you don't want to let that person down, it's harder to give up and quit.

A health club will also offer ways to help you stick to it, whether in an aerobics class or on a stationary bicycle. By going regularly to the same health club, you'll develop new acquaintances. You'll begin to establish a camaraderie with many people with similar goals. And most of them want to have a good time, too.

The Buddy System helps you put into practice what most professional athletes discover in training years—no athletic successes are ever achieved alone. You always need the assistance of someone else training you, encouraging you and motivating you.

If sticking to the program becomes a burden, perhaps you are striving for too much too soon. You may need to re-evaluate your short-term goals and, if necessary, rewrite them. If taking several days off from exercise is what you need to remain on your program, then do it. Exercise should not be punishment. It should be a small vacation from your daily routine—a vacation that offers you a change and a physical and emotional release from daily activities.

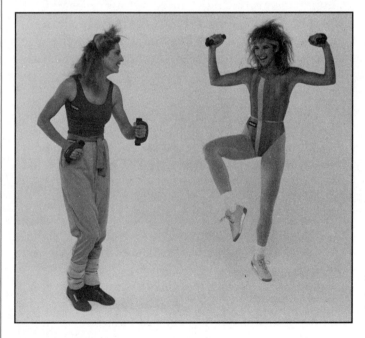

The Buddy System works even if you and your buddy aren't at the same level of fitness.

We can't encourage you enough to stick to it because there *is* a point of no return. Eventually you realize that not only do you want to exercise but you want to encourage others to do the same. You'll find that the Buddy System ends up meaning that everyone who exercises is your buddy.

Prepare Yourself Emotionally—This is what you need most to get through the initial stages of starting out. In addition, it will offer you the training needed to remain on a program and make fitness a way of life.

The mental approach to any exercise program is much more important than most people realize. Mental processes must be trained, too. According to one scientist, "We can only speculate how much athletes who do not realize their potential are held back by personal factors other than skill and conditioning . . . Athletes must either activate or relax thought processes to ready themselves for competition."

The mind can be trained to do one of two things for you when you exercise—it can take your attention away from the experience or it can intensify the attention you give to the activity. Even though you made the commitment, your body has to feel it, too. And that takes relaxation of mind and body.

Deep-breathing exercises are useful for relaxation. If you are tense or emotionally upset, your breath comes in short pants from the top of the rib cage. By breathing deep from the diaphragm, you can create an opposite effect. Place your hands at the bottom of the rib cage so that the fingers of both hands lightly touch. Take a deep breath, pulling the air into the diaphragm so that your fingers are drawn apart as the diaphragm swells. Do this three or four times.

We suggest that you incorporate relaxation exercises in your MuscleAerobics program. Use them as a mild warm-up at the beginning or as an effective cool-down after a strenuous workout. Stretching exercises are also particularly relaxing if not performed too vigorously.

STEP 5: GET READY NUTRITIONALLY

Studies have shown that regular exercise plays an important role in maintaining, enhancing and restoring health. But is exercise the only ingredient necessary to stay healthy? No, nutrition is the missing link. Combining good nutrition with a healthy, physically fit body is working with your body both inside and out. One is lost without the other.

Let's consider the definition of *health*. The word is derived from the Anglo-Saxon word *haelth,* meaning the condition of being safe and sound, or whole. For many years this historical concept was ignored. Health was merely viewed as freedom from disease.

An essential way to create an overall condition of health is to develop good eating habits. Even so, you may see or hear of successful athletes eating candy bars, fast foods, soda and other non-nutritious foods. How can this be?

Basically, it's similar to the performance difference in your car when you use regular gasoline instead of high-octane gasoline, or a low-grade motor oil instead of a quality motor oil. Of course the car will run, especially if you keep up maintenance. But really caring for your car both inside and out will make it run as smoothly as it possibly can.

Your body acts in almost the same way, because the amounts and kinds of food you eat determine body size, endurance, strength and performance. If you desire success in any program, you must follow a proper diet, whether it's a weight-loss program or not.

To be well-nourished, two requirements must be met. Food not only provides energy, but also the raw materials for new tissue and metabolic functions. Even when food intake is balanced to meet all bodily needs, the exercise level affects the use of the various nutrients. For example, strenuous exercise, like Muscle Aerobics, creates metabolic needs different from resting needs.

Nutrients in food are usually classified six ways—water, minerals, vitamins, proteins, fats and carbohydrates.

Water—An adequate supply of water is essential. Although you can survive quite a few days without food, you cannot survive long without water. It is your aid for temperature control at rest and during exercise. It helps transport the nutrients to your cells and is necessary for elimination.

Minerals—Some minerals, such as sodium, potassium and chlorine, are part of

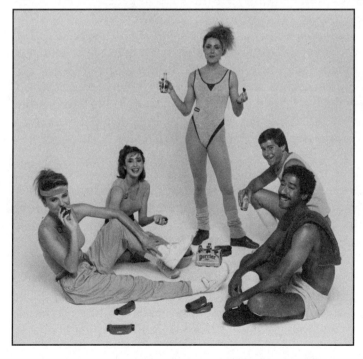

You must consider good nutrition as part of any fitness lifestyle. Between shooting sessions for this book, our models snacked on Perrier mineral water, California figs and other healthful foods.

physical work. They maintain a proper balance of fluids, and are also significant for impulse transmission along nervous and muscular membranes.

Other minerals, such as calcium, phosphorus and magnesium, are essential for health, including dental and bone formation. Certain trace minerals are needed for normal growth, tissue repair and blood cell formation.

Iron is a most important mineral, especially for women. It helps produce new hemoglobin, a protein substance in blood that creates the red color and carries oxygen. In this sense, iron is highly needed for endurance and physical performance.

Vitamins—These are organic substances that regulate chemical reactions. Vitamins contribute to growth and the maintenance of life. Because vitamins are only slightly involved with body structure and offer a limited supply of energy for body functions, vitamin needs among athletes and nonathletes are about the same. Therefore, it isn't necessary to consume more than the recommended dosage.

Fats—As mentioned earlier, fat is not bad in itself. When too much food is consumed, the excess is stored as fat. Needless to say, when this is the case, your physical performance is affected, not to mention your health. But fats are an important energy source, especially during aerobic exercise. Fats also insulate you from extreme temperature. And when combined with cholesterol, fat is involved in the formation of cell membranes.

The important thing we must emphasize is that fats in general act as an effective fuel source. The problem fat is *excess fat*. The excess stays in your fat cells and only make you look fat.

Carbohydrates—The basic unit of carbohydrates is the simple sugar, glucose. As explained earlier, sugars in such foods as honey, fruits and breads are all absorbed by your gastrointestinal tract and consequently changed to glucose. Much of the glucose is passed into the blood and transported to the body tissues and muscles. The amount of glucose available is gradually reduced unless some form of carbohydrate is eaten during the day. So when you're exercising, the supply gets depleted rapidly.

According to the Department of Nutrition at Harvard University, there is evidence that endurance sports require a diet high in complex carbohydrates. Research seems to indicate that complex carbohydrates significantly improve performance. In addition, it has been determined that carbohydrates should provide over 50% of your total caloric intake if you participate in these types of programs.

Don't confuse carbohydrates with fatty foods, though. You may have heard the expression *carbo-loading* from runners who compete in races. The night before a race they eat seemingly anything and everything—pizza, cookies, ice cream and many other sugared creations. They are not carbo-loading; they

The Active Athlete's Nutrition Plan

1) Always eat a good breakfast.

2) Nutritionists are discovering that five smaller meals a day are better for some people than three larger ones. Better digestion usually results.

3) No more junk foods. In general, they are empty calories.

4) Snack on fresh vegetables and fruit.

5) Don't eat the same foods every day. Variety helps create a nutritional balance and ensures maximum intake of nutrients.

6) Check your diet regularly. Consider keeping a nutritional chart to make sure that you are eating foods from all food groups.

7) Avoid fatty foods, especially before a workout, because they slow digestion.

8) Minimize consumption of red meat. Instead, eat more poultry, fish and vegetable proteins.

9) Drink plenty of water. It is the athlete's most important beverage. Drink a minimum of eight glasses per day.

10) Consume one cup of milk or yogurt daily.

11) Eat whole-grain breads and cereals instead of products made with bleached, white flour.

12) Eat fresh fruit daily.

13) Eat at least four helpings of vegetables daily. Include both dark-green vegetables (such as spinach) and yellow vegetables (such as carrots).

14) Avoid "chemical-type" additives such as saccharin, cyclamates and monosodium glutamate.

15) Reduce salt intake.

16) Eat balanced calories: Carbohydrates 60% to 70%, Protein 15% to 20%, Fats 10% to 15%. Complex carbohydrates provide the athlete with what's needed most—energy. These include: grains, breads, potatoes.

17) Supplement your diet with vitamins, but don't take megadoses.

18) Eat in a relaxed, enjoyable environment.

19) Try not to eat after 6:00 p.m. Or, eat very lightly after that time.

20) Don't eat right before or after a workout. Eat no less than two hours before a workout and wait at least one hour after working out before eating.

are fat-loading. When we say include over 50% carbohydrates in your diet, we're talking about complex carbohydrates. These are low-fat, high-fiber carbohydrates, such as unprocessed fruits, grains and vegetables. Without a doubt, MuscleAerobics is a high-endurance sport. You should consider this type of diet.

Proteins—The basic elements of proteins are amino acids. Proteins form the structural parts of cells, hormones, enzymes and muscle molecules. Protein concentration varies, however. For example, muscle has about 20% protein, and nerve tissue has about 10% protein.

The variety of proteins needed by various body cells requires a source of amino acids. The only common foods that have *all* of the essential amino acids are soybeans and meat. Therefore, you will need to supplement your diet with different types of protein foods to ensure that you are receiving all of the necessary amino acids.

Some people, such as weightlifters, think that they need to consume lots of protein—more than their bodies can use. But because amino acids can't be stored by the body, much of the excess is passed in urine. Most of the energy you need is supplied by fats and carbohydrates and little, if any, protein. Increasing your intake of protein by eating steaks, raw eggs and protein drinks won't make you stronger.

Balanced Diet—Nutrition doesn't have to be complicated. In fact, dividing foods into four major groups is the best way we know to make nutrition really simple. You've probably heard of them before, and nutritionally, not much has changed since. Basically the four groups are meat, fruits and vegetables, bread and whole grains, and dairy products.

The meat group includes red meat, poultry, fish, eggs, peanuts and other protein sources such as soybeans. The other categories are self-explanatory. The basic habit of three meals a day still holds true, but some people actually prefer *five* smaller meals a day.

When to Eat—Don't cheat yourself nutritionally by skipping meals. Eating one huge meal per day creates a poor nutritional cycle. In addition, research indicates that it is probably best to eat your largest meal at midday. Dr. Kenneth Cooper writes, "If you consume the largest proportion of your calories *before* 1:00 p.m., you will have less of a problem controlling your weight than if you consume the same number of calories *after* 1:00 p.m."

Dr. Kenneth Cooper believes that by taking in most of your food early in the day, you can process it more readily. The assumption is that your body remains relatively active during most of the digestive process. This makes sense because most people are not very active after 5:00 or 8:00 p.m. Also, it's known that the body's metabolism tends to increase during the early part of the day and then slow down toward evening.

This can mean that you burn fewer calories in the evening than earlier in the day. But remember, exercise increases metabolism. By exercising in the late afternoon, you may increase your metabolic rate and in turn that can increase calorie burning in the evening.

Either way, you need to exercise regularly and eat a balanced diet. The only thing to add here is that you should eat two hours before you exercise and wait at least an hour before eating after you exercise.

STEP 6: PREVENTING EXERCISE BURNOUT

Almost everyone has experienced exercise burnout of some kind. Typically, this happens because you wanted to accomplish too much too fast. How about those aerobic classes you were taking every day for weeks and finally you didn't want to go any more at all? You were frustrated; you couldn't keep up; and you felt exhausted all the time.

You probably blamed the instructor, as most people do when starting out. This is human. We always find someone or something to blame when we want to give up.

But don't despair. Remember that fitness is a way of life. Maintaining a fit lifestyle is a continual process. By pushing yourself too far and too fast, you may find yourself right back where you started.

Have Fun—The secret to enjoying exercise is simple. First, you need to understand what kind of exercise will produce the most benefits for you. And you already know the answer to that—MuscleAerobics!

The next thing you need to understand is to exercise slowly and gradually. We've said this already, and we'll continue to say it.

If your excuse for quitting is exhaustion, don't blame it on the exercise leader. If he or she is doing a fast-paced run for 20 minutes and you can only jog or just lift your feet slightly off the ground, then just jog and be proud. Don't worry. In time you'll be able to run instead of jog for those 20 minutes.

Although MuscleAerobics is a sport, it is not a competitive sport. If you must compete, compete with yourself at your own pace. You can't expect the aerobics instructor to slow down the class for you. You can control your own pace.

Pacing—Whatever you do, don't come to a complete stop. Just slow down. Concentrate on your breathing and how your body feels. Part of getting in shape is training your body to stay in motion for at least 30 minutes at a time. So don't quit moving. Slow down or do whatever it takes to stay with the routine.

Of course, once you can sustain MuscleAerobics for at least 30 minutes, you can go on and push yourself a little harder. But remember, even though you may be breathing hard during MuscleAerobics, you shouldn't be working so hard that you get out of breath and can't talk. Then exhaustion and thoughts of quitting set in.

By overtraining, you can overtax your body in more ways than just muscle breakdown. Pushing yourself too hard and too fast can lead to injury.

Here are two ways to monitor whether you are overtraining or not—keep track of your resting pulse rate and weight. Take your pulse before you rise every morning or at least every other morning. If it's up 5 to 10 beats from the day before, either decrease your workout for that day or don't work out at all. Weigh yourself at about the same time each day. Large fluctuations mean that you're working out too hard. We might also add, getting less sleep than usual contributes to muscle fatigue.

Once your body adapts to MuscleAerobics, you'll know how hard to push yourself. Some days you'll have so much energy, you'll feel like "pushing to the edge." Other days you may want to coast through the workout. But that's OK, too.

We did say that you need to exercise at least five days a week to achieve weight loss, but five days a week may be your burnout level. So at first, don't try to workout everyday. Every other day is fine at first. Give your body a chance to rest in between. And when you get stronger, you can increase the workouts.

CHAPTER FIVE

Muscle-Aerobics Technique

Sports psychologist Bruce Ogilvie sees today's fitness phenomenon as "putting one's body and talent on trial." Olympic athletes may have more talent, but not necessarily greater dedication than the rest of us. With this dedication we are looking to attain our personal best.

To that end, all top athletes know that one way to achieve excellence is through proper technique. We everyday athletes are no different. For safety and athletic achievement, nothing counts as much as proper technique.

Some people train with a daily workout to become technically better at their sport. Others rely on their sport strictly to get them in shape. The "fitter" person, the one who includes training for the sport and practices the sport, will almost always win over the less fit or "weekend athlete."

Despite the obvious differences in focus, there is a common thread binding together sports conditioning and fitness training. Sports conditioning will enable you to get in shape and excel in your particular sport. Fitness training will get you in shape to play *any* sport.

To become stronger, have more endurance, or acquire more flexibility, you must place your body under physical stress of some sort. The most common method is fitness training, based on weight training, basic calisthenics and aerobic-type exercises. MuscleAerobics offers this type of fitness training in one type of workout. For both general fitness and general sports conditioning, MuscleAerobics is extremely productive.

BEFORE STARTING

We define *technique* as proper application of form, ability and flexibility. In most sports, technique—including how you position your body or hold equipment—is important in experiencing success. MuscleAerobics is no different.

Athletic Oneness—To experience success in any sport—whether tennis, skiing, ice skating or even pingpong—athletes must first learn to "become one" with their equipment. This technique makes the equipment feel like a natural extension of the body. Oneness is most often the result of proper body positioning, which leads in turn to proper execution.

To follow this logic, remember the first time you tried to ride a two-wheel bike. When you rode a tricycle or a bike with training wheels, it didn't matter much how you sat on the bike or how you rode. But when you tried a two-wheeler, you had to figure out effective body positioning so you could balance the bicycle.

When you began to feel balanced, you may have been able to ride for a while but probably with some trepidation. But the remaining fear disappeared as you began to feel more in control. Eventually, your sense of balance harmonized with your basic coordination and you became "one" with your bicycle. Today, it's easy to tell when a child senses this oneness because he starts doing daredevil "wheelies" all over the neighborhood.

In a sport such as tennis, top women's pro Martina Navratilova beautifully displays her perfect form when she executes a shot. She deftly maneuvers the racket as a controlled extension of her arm and hand.

But Navratilova didn't always have her current form and consistency. An article in *The Physician and Sports Medicine* (June 1984) discusses Martina's early pro career and her somewhat undisciplined training routine. For example, she was known for going horseback riding the day before a major tournament, instead of resting, practicing or concentrating on the upcoming match. She made the transition from tennis star to tennis champion when she combined her natural ability with a program to develop herself as a total athlete.

To effectively participate in a MuscleAerobics program, you need similar attentiveness. Body positioning is important. You also need to make the weights beneficial extensions of your arms and hands. Eventually, you will be training as a total athlete—developing flexibility, strength, endurance, coordination, poise and balance.

Safety Through Technique—Any type of strenuous exercise will submit your body to possible muscle strains or tears. Proper MuscleAerobics technique will help you avoid potential muscle strains and tears.

Proper technique in this sense involves pacing yourself and listening to your body signals. Pacing yourself can mean anything from determining your fitness level to starting gradually and then easing off during times of fatigue. Listening to body signals will allow you to progress with comfort, not strain. It will prevent you from pushing too hard and, in turn, help you to push only when you're ready. Listening to body signals will also help keep away the ''put-it-off-until-tomorrow syndrome'' caused by exercise burnout.

WHERE TO START

In the previous chapter you got some physical and mental advice and determined whether you should begin MuscleAerobics at the beginning, intermediate or advanced level.

Next, you need to determine the amount of weight you are capable of handling. An easy way to analyze the proper amount of weight is by using a pair of one-pound weights in a controlled pumping action without stopping during your aerobics class. If you find that you have to stop or that movements become uncontrollable due to the weight, either use a smaller weight or start your program on a stationary bicycle.

The MuscleAerobics exercises in this book are designed so a beginner can move right into a program with ease. However, no matter how advanced you are aerobically, adding any weight will affect your workout. MuscleAerobics requires good aerobic capacity coupled with the necessary muscular strength to handle light weights during active aerobic exercise.

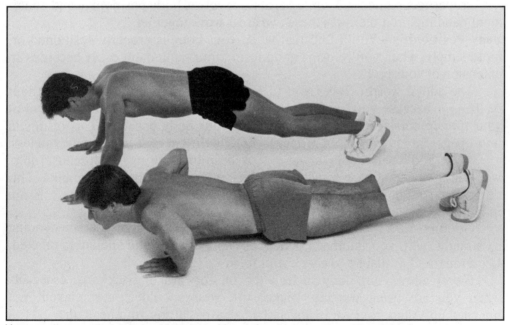

You may discover that you shouldn't start a MuscleAerobics program with weights because you aren't yet strong enough. If that's the case, we recommend that you increase upper-body strength by doing pushups, as described in the text.

If You Aren't Strong Enough to Start with Weights — As discussed before, one of the best ways to increase upper body strength *without* using weights is by doing pushups. The method we endorse is a *slow,* four-count movement: On the way down, count, "one one-thousand, two one-thousand, three one-thousand, four one-thousand." On the way up count, "one one-thousand, two one-thousand."

Make sure that your chest is just touching the floor when you reach the down count of "four one-thousand." If you find that doing one set is strenuous, start off by keeping your knees bent. Do three sets of 8 to 12 repetitions every day for about a month. Also, continue with your aerobics class.

Work toward eventually doing the pushups with legs straight for added resistance. You'll soon notice that the slow, controlled movements will build strength in your arms, chest and back muscles.

Caution: If you are over 35 years of age and have not exercised regularly for more than 6 to 12 months, we recommend that you discuss an alternate set of strength-building exercises with your physician.

BASIC MUSCLEAEROBICS TECHNIQUE

When you have the minimum strength requirements, you're ready for the MuscleAerobics challenge.

Proper technique for MuscleAerobics involves body positioning and equipment handling. In most cases these two areas work together.

Body Positioning — You'll find that when your body is properly positioned or, more simply, when you're using good form, your equipment easily becomes an extension of your body.

The added weight forces you to become aware of body position without realizing it because you have to *control* the movements. If you lose control of your movements, you also lose control of your body position. This results in improper technique. Without proper technique the exercise will benefit you less.

Your body will be in a variety of positions during a MuscleAerobics workout. On a stationary bicycle, you'll have the secure base of the bike. This doesn't mean, however, that body positioning on a stationary bicycle is not important.

Good posture is critical. For floor exercises, be sure that you are standing up straight, with your stomach pulled in, chest uplifted and shoulders relaxed. Use a mirror, if available, to check your form.

Never allow your body to lean too far forward or backward, especially when you are using weights. Make sure your shoulders are relaxed, not hunched up. Allow yourself to feel as if a balloon is lifting your head up.

Following these tips will help you maintain a relaxed, erect position. As you gain upper-body strength your spinal cord will be better protected by the

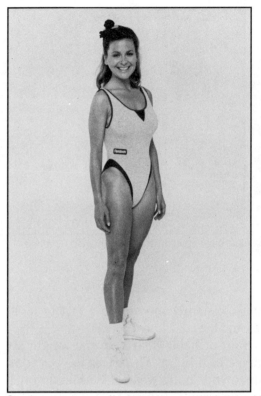 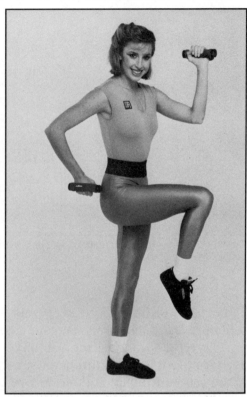

Good posture pays off even when you aren't doing MuscleAerobics.

toned muscles in your back. Stronger muscles mean a greater ability to defy gravity and hold the body erect. An uplifted, erect posture provides greater lung capacity and also allows other organs to operate at greater efficiency. Also, your muscles will tend to move with ease, resulting in better coordination.

Weak upper-body muscles lead to a slouched posture. Among other things, poor posture puts additional stress on certain muscles and organs, causing the lungs and heart to work harder. In short, a weak upper body means that your upper torso muscles work harder and produce fewer benefits.

Foot Placement—Knees should always remain slightly bent or in a relaxed position whether you are standing or running. Locked knees strain ligaments and put pressure on the joints.

Make sure your knees are always supported by squarely-placed feet. Be sure that your weight is evenly distributed.

Don't put unnecessary stress on your knees, ankles and feet by hopping or jumping on one foot for extended periods of time before switching feet. In other words, alternate your kicks from foot to foot.

At first, keep your feet relatively close to the floor, moving them faster

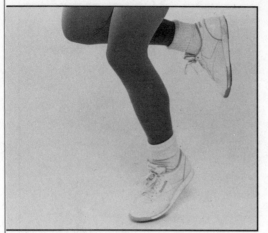 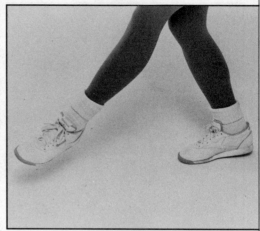

Don't hop on one foot for more than four counts. The ideal movement is an alternating hop from one foot to the other, as above.

rather than higher. If you keep your feet constantly moving to a fast beat, it helps prevent undue stress on your ankles and legs.

Never land on just the ball of your foot or heel. Distribute the weight so that your foot is going through its full range of motion. The stress to your foot when you're running is three to five times your body weight. With additional weights, this can increase to 10 times your weight. Proper foot placement is very important.

Body Alignment on a Stationary Bicycle—Adjust the bike seat to suit your height and leg length. When sitting on the bike, extend your right leg straight down and rest your foot on the pedal in its lowest (6 o'clock) position. If you can hardly reach the pedal, the seat is too high.

Adjust the seat so body weight is firmly balanced on the seat and the ball of your right foot is resting on the pedal. As shown in the photo on page 33 and those of chapter 6 your right leg should have a slightly bent knee.

Relaxed but Firm Arms—Any time you work a body part, work up to a full range of motion. For example, when running in place, eventually pick up your feet and completely bend the knees. Work the whole leg.

Arms should either swing or pump with full extension, starting with a bent elbow. When the movement requires arm straightening, don't partially straighten the arm. Take the arm through the full range of motion.

The same applies with the bent elbow. Bend the elbow completely. By partially straightening the arm or partially bending the elbow, you are shortening muscle. Always fully extend and contract the muscles you are working. This will help you maintain complete flexibility in the working muscles.

Relaxed but Firm Grip—The weights should be secured just enough so they don't fly out of your hand. Don't overgrip them. This will create undue muscle tension.

About every five minutes, wiggle your fingers to relax your grip. Long distance cyclists are told to move their hands every few minutes on the handlebars to prevent cramping and possible nerve-pinching. The same advice applies to handweights of any sort. When relaxing your grip, slow down the arm movement. Then open and close fingers in succession and wiggle them.

Keep Arms Moving—The key to a MuscleAerobics program is combining upper- and lower-body movements. When you move your arms, be sure to exert some type of pumping action. Don't let your arms dangle at your side. Movements should be controlled—never choppy or swinging out of control.

Try to relate the pumping action of your arms to the pumping of your heart. As you start to fatigue, slow down foot movements, not arm movements.

Work Muscle—When pumping or pushing with weights, concentrate on this: The strength of the movement comes from your shoulders and arms.

There is a tendency to create movement based on momentum rather than muscle. Such a pendulum effect merely keeps your body moving, rather than working the specific muscles that are waiting to benefit.

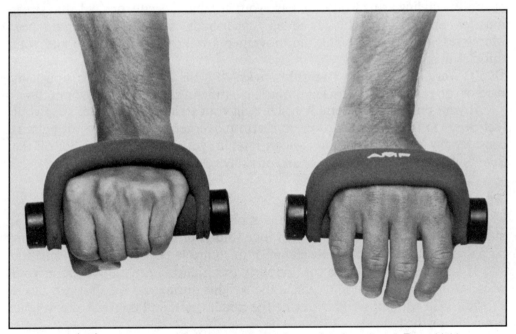

Overgripping (left) causes unnecessary muscle tension in your hands and arms. To avoid this, periodically relax your grip and wiggle your fingers (right). Some handweights, such as the Heavyhands shown here, are designed so overgripping is not much of a problem. There's more about available handweights in chapter 7.

Use the Right Handweights—Whether you do MuscleAerobics in an aerobics class or on a stationary bicycle, you'll need the right weight for the setting. In chapter 7, we discuss the different weights available for a MuscleAerobics program.

Size of weight, fit and comfort are very important. When using steel or smooth-textured weights, be careful as you perspire. Sweat can make the weights slippery.

ADDITIONAL PRECAUTIONS

With almost every benefit, there is an accompanying precaution or guideline. Here we want to stress some of the more important cautions. Keeping these points in mind will put you on the road to a safe, injury-free MuscleAerobics program.

Start with Light Weights—When in doubt, start with weights that are too light rather than too heavy. In this case, more is not better.

Control is the key. Don't risk the possibility of injury by using heavier weight when your upper body is trying to adjust to the added resistance.

Don't Use Choppy Motions—Always continue the movement through your full range of motion. By shortening the movement, you will lose the full benefit. Dangling arms won't increase your aerobic capacity, nor will you stress muscles enough to achieve added upper-body strength and endurance. Moreover, actions shortening the movements will cause you to tire and your muscles to cramp rapidly.

Don't Work to Extreme Breathlessness—If your breathing feels unusually hard or too easy during MuscleAerobics, it's time to stop and check your pulse.

If your pulse is considerably faster than your training heart rate, keep your feet closer to the floor and lower your arm movements slightly. If your pulse is considerably below your training heart rate, lift your feet slightly higher off the floor and pump your arms higher and possibly more vigorously.

ABOUT MUSCLE FATIGUE

MuscleAerobics is an endurance sport, and as any sport requiring real stamina, muscle fatigue is a factor. Move into your program carefully, making sure that fatigue does not create sloppy or uncontrolled upper body movements.

If you find that you are continuously experiencing muscle fatigue in your MuscleAerobics programs, try using the weights during just the first part of the program. Go without weights during the middle part, and then use the weights again during the last part.

Try to use the weights a little longer each time during this type of program. But don't be discouraged if you don't progress right away. Pay attention to your body signals. Your body will let you know when you're ready.

MUSCLEAEROBICS IN ACTION

Dr. Leonard Schwartz, the author of *Heavyhands,* endorses three primary levels when working with weights. In the beginning level, the weights are confined to movements below the waist. In the intermediate level, the weights are lifted to the waist and slightly above. And in the advanced level, the weights are lifted to shoulder height and above.

Although the MuscleAerobics program incorporates all three stages in a variety of routines, more emphasis on arm height will be placed at the appropriate stage. For example, an advanced MuscleAerobics class uses *more* moves above the shoulders than at other levels. According to Dr. Schwartz, a heavy weight lifted to a height of one foot, at the same pace, could produce as much oxygen consumption as a much lighter weight at a height of three feet.

The kind of stress you apply to your body will determine your eventual fitness. Therefore, it is critical to understand your fitness level and know which weights and intensity levels are best for you. Once you have mastered the weights, you can make certain variations that yield significant improvements with little or no extra effort.

How to Progress—To progress, you should increase the stress in one of three ways: 1) by adding more weight, 2) exercising longer, or 3) increasing the intensity of your program.

As you recall, increased workouts will mean exercising more than three times per week. Five times per week will provide weight loss and fitness-level progression. But perhaps all you have time for is three times a week. In this case, our suggestion is to consider increasing the weight and the amount of time you workout for those three days. Obviously, we've designed practicality and convenience into our MuscleAerobics program.

Occasional breaks or days off from exercising are needed to avoid overtraining. If you apply too much stress, as in too much exercising day after day, you can throw your body into *exhaustion.* Overtraining results in diminished returns in your progressive workout. You will start to go backward instead of forward. The only real cure for overtraining is to decrease your workout.

To avoid exhaustion, start exercising gradually, easing through the initial stages. Then slowly intensify the workout until you reach your desired level.

If the content, intensity and duration of MuscleAerobics remain the same, your body will adapt and improvement will cease. A good way to progress is to start by using two-pound handweights on a stationary bicycle on Tuesdays and Thursdays and one-pound handweights in an aerobics classes on Mondays, Wednesdays and Fridays.

This kind of schedule will allow you to slowly introduce additional weight into your program. Your body can then slowly adjust to this new stress and adapt so you can eventually use the two-pound handweights every day.

TECHNIQUE AND SPORTS ETIQUETTE

In addition to technique, each sport has its own etiquette. For example, in tennis and racquetball you do not wear black-soled shoes. Games such as basketball and football have penalties to ensure some etiquette.

Most etiquette evolves from the need for courtesy and safety. MuscleAerobics has etiquette, too.

You must maintain proper distance from your fellow MuscleAerobic partners. Before using the weights, look around, hold your arms straight out at your sides, then turn and make a complete circle. This shows if anyone is in your way. The last thing you want to do is "bonk" someone on the head as she works alongside you trying to get fit.

MuscleAerobics on a stationary bicycle also requires certain courtesies. Make sure your arm movements don't swing back too far—there might be a person or mirror directly behind you.

More Essential Points

Our main message in this book is that you should develop a lifestyle that embraces fitness. To that end, your fitness routine should be as follows:

1) Fun.
2) Realistic.
3) Able to fit into your daily routine.
4) Challenging without being too stressful.
5) Accomplished in a time frame you can commit to.
6) Progressive, allowing you the ability to develop safely.
7) Practical both indoors and outdoors.
8) Goal-oriented to help you lose weight, gain strength, improve flexibility and increase endurance.

It is our firm belief that MuscleAerobics does all of that. For best results, be sure to follow our recommendations in the book. Our research and tests prove that they work.

We also urge you to consult your physician before beginning *any* exercise program, but especially before starting MuscleAerobics. It can only help you achieve what you are physically able to accomplish. Your doctor's advice should precede any program.

When you have the "green light," then move on with confidence. A fitness lifestyle will help you enter a whole new world of friendships, vitality and (we hope) a longer, happier life.

CHAPTER SIX

Muscle-Aerobics Fitness Menu

Using weights for strength training or for bodybuilding is becoming an increasingly popular form of conditioning for both men and women. Without proper instruction, however, it's easy to damage muscles, bones and joints.

10 COMMON MISTAKES

Mike Mentzer, the only person to win the Mr. Universe title with a perfect score, has identified 10 training mistakes commonly made by people using weights. We've been sure to incorporate his advice into MuscleAerobics. Here are some general ways to avoid problems:

1) Overtraining—Train hard *or* long, but not hard *and* long.

2) Lack of Intensity—The beneficial effects of MuscleAerobics happen when you neither overexert nor underexert.

3) Sloppy Performance—Slow, steady movements using correct form produce results.

4) Poor Warmup/Poor Cooldown—Skipping either one or both will probably save time, but it will also make you susceptible to injury.

5) Muscle Imbalance—Train every part of the body with equal intensity to avoid muscle imbalances.

6) Excess Weight—Don't use weights that are too heavy. Know your limits.

7) Breathing—Pay attention to proper breathing while exercising.

8) Poor Nutrition—Maintain a balanced, sensible diet.

9) Overeating—Don't increase your caloric intake just because you're working out more.

10) Poor Attitude—Give your workouts a worthwhile direction. Unrealistic goals only set the stage for failure.

YOUR FITNESS MENU

In previous chapters we've discussed what the body needs and how it moves. This information will help you develop a program that is suited to achieving your personal potential. Before jumping into your program, take time to explore proper technique and review the do's and don'ts of MuscleAerobics in chapter 5. With this background knowledge, you have all of the guidelines you need to create a MuscleAerobics program that works for you.

Essentials—When creating a program, remember the following fitness goals: endurance, strength, coordination, balance, flexibility and body awareness. All should be incorporated into a program that includes exercises in this order: warmup, stretch, aerobic work, cooldown and stretch.

A well-balanced MuscleAerobics program requires specific attention to all aspects of body conditioning. Proper preparation is as important as doing the activity itself. For this reason, we have created a "Fitness Menu" of exercises that offers you an enjoyable 30- to 60-minute program of MuscleAerobics. We also suggest a few general exercises for warming up, stretching and cooling down. These are highly recommended to all MuscleAerobic participants, whether you're at a beginner, intermediate or advanced level.

Warmup and Cooldown—You should begin any exercise program with a warmup and end it with a cooldown. For MuscleAerobics we recommend that

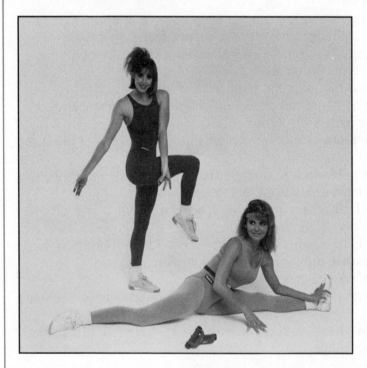

As explained in the text, warmup, stretching and cooldown are important. Don't neglect them!

you use weights during the aerobic portion only—not during the warmup, cool-down and stretching exercises.

Warming up and cooling down are essential transitions between activity and inactivity. A warmup will progressively stimulate the heart and lungs, increase blood flow and gradually increase the muscle and blood temperatures. In addition, a complete warmup will stretch muscles in preparation for a more strenuous workout.

Don't do warmup exercises fast or with jerky movements. They can create possible tendon or muscle tears and ruptures. Use active, controlled movements.

After you have sufficiently warmed the muscles, follow with static or slow stretching, not bouncing movements. Stretching is an easy and relaxing way to prepare for exercise, as shown later in this chapter. In other words, stretching should never be stressful. Each individual has his or her own muscular structure and varying tension levels. Damage to the ligaments can often be traced to improper stretching techniques and overstretching.

Remember to consciously focus on the muscle you are stretching. Try to relax that part. Always breathe deeply and regularly while stretching. Never hold your breath.

Aerobics—Once you have warmed up and stretched muscles, you are ready to begin the aerobics portion. Now it's time to pick up your MuscleAerobic weights and begin jogging in place or hop on the stationary bicycle.

Remember that to achieve endurance, you have to meet three requirements: frequency, intensity and duration. Start slowly, building up to a steady, uninterrupted activity for at least 20 minutes. Ideally, 30 minutes at your training heart rate is best.

Because steady activity is important, don't substantially increase and decrease the intensity of your movements. Doubling the amount of exercise will not necessarily double its effects. Intensified efforts may cause chronically sore muscles—an indication of overworked muscles.

Cooldown—Just as you slowly increase the intensity of your aerobic movements when beginning a workout, you need to slowly decrease the intensity when ending it. Never bring any aerobic activity to an abrupt end.

For example, if you were running in place, you would bring the body down to a slow jog and then possibly reduce to a brisk march or walking movement before stretching your muscles. Allowing your body to cooldown slowly will let your muscles effectively assist in pumping blood from the arms and legs back to the heart. If you end your run abruptly, your heart will continue to send extra blood to the muscles for a few more minutes.

Because you are no longer working the muscles at this point and helping to direct the blood back to the heart, blood may pool into the muscles. This may result in insufficient blood for other parts of the body. In fact, if you don't keep moving, you may experience dizziness. Stretching exercises should always follow the warmup and cooldown segments.

WARMUP EXERCISES (10 MINUTES)

Begin your warmup exercises by standing erect with your feet shoulder-width apart. Maintain good posture by expanding your chest, relaxing your shoulders, holding in your abdomen and tucking in the buttocks. Do these exercises with at least 8 to 12 repetitions unless instructed otherwise. Warmups should be vigorous enough to increase your breathing and heart rate slightly.

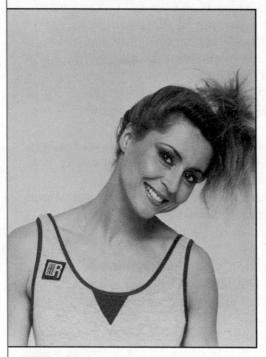 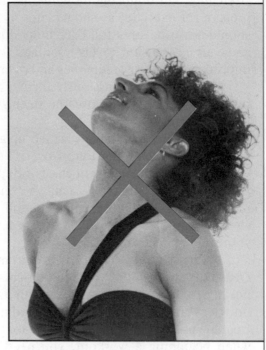

HEAD ROLLS
Gently and slowly roll your head to the right shoulder and then over to the left shoulder, as shown in the photo at left. Do four repetitions. Do not drop your head back, as shown at right.

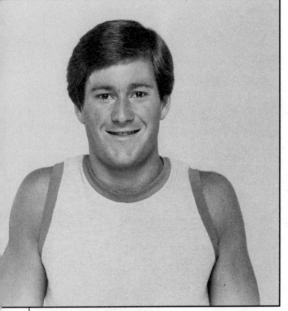 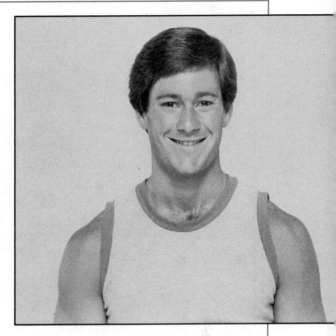

SHOULDER SHRUGS
Stand with your arms hanging loosely at your sides. Raise your shoulders up to your ears, then relax and press them as far down as possible. Do four repetitions.
   Here's a variation: Roll the shoulders all the way forward then roll them all the way back.

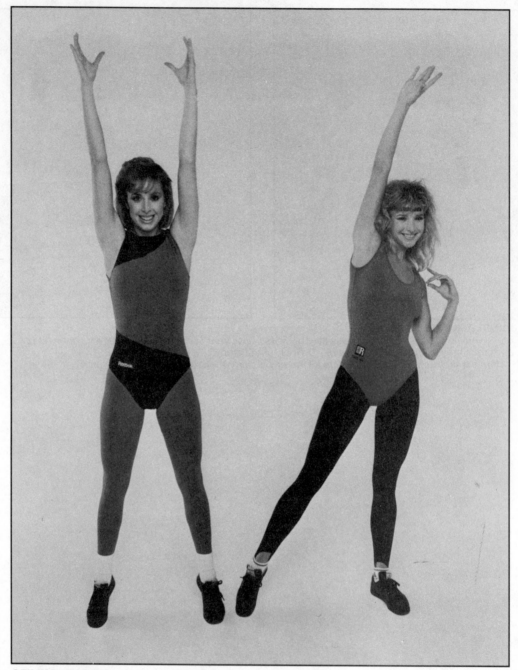

CEILING REACHES
Stand with both arms reaching straight overhead. Pretend that you are trying to touch the ceiling. Alternately reach the left arm up, bending the left knee at the same time. Then reach with the right arm up, bending the right knee at the same time. Do 10 repetitions.

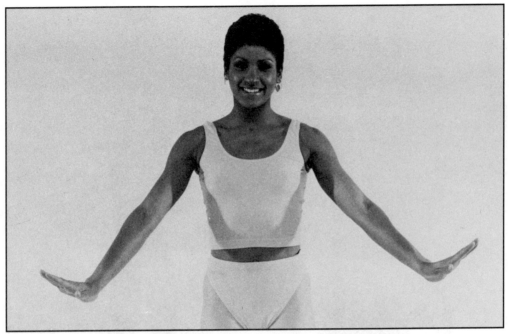

ARM CIRCLES
Hold both arms straight out sideways, slightly below shoulder level. Form small circling movements, gradually getting larger. Reverse direction. Do five repetitions in each direction.

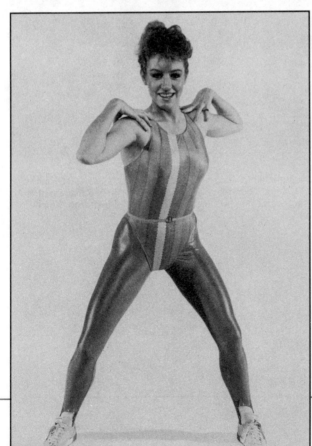

TRUNK TWISTS
Hold your arms at shoulder height with your hands resting on your shoulders. Twist your upper body alternately from side to side. Keep your back straight and your knees slightly bent. At each twist, try to look as far over your shoulder as possible without moving your hips. Do 12 repetitions.

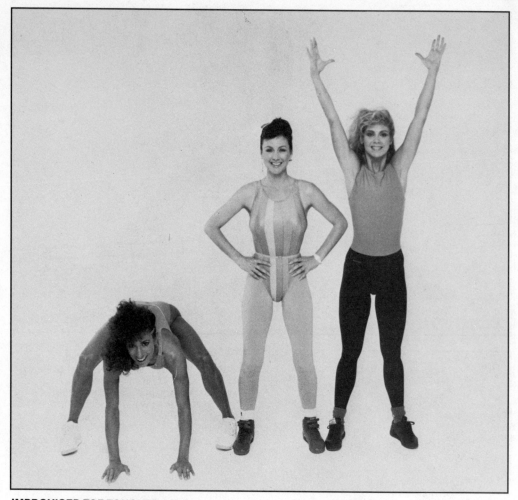

IMPROVISED TOE TOUCHES
Stand erect with both arms reaching toward the ceiling. Next, place both hands at your waist. Finally touch your toes, keeping your knees bent. From the floor, place your hands on your waist again, then reach back to the ceiling. The order is: ceiling-waist-floor-waist-ceiling. This is one stretch. Do not pause between counts. Do eight repetitions.

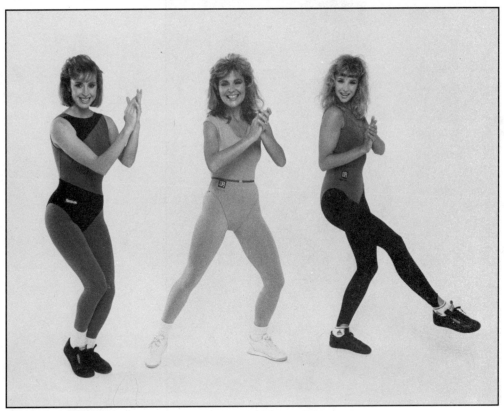

SIDE-TO-SIDE SHUFFLE
Step from side to side, clapping your hands with each step. You may want to vary the stepping movement to alternate leg kicks without bouncing. Do 12 to 15 repetitions.

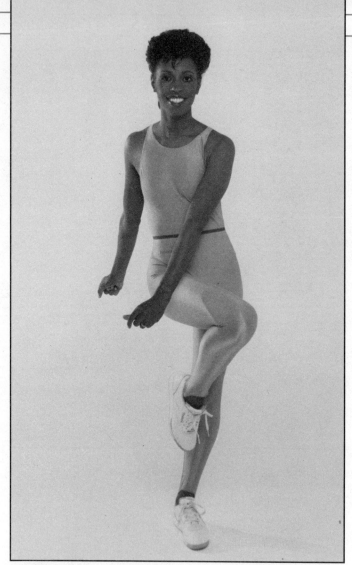

ALTERNATE BENT-KNEE LIFTS
Bend the right knee and raise it up close to waist height. Repeat with
the other knee. Do not bounce or jump. Do 8 to 12 repetitions.

STRETCHING EXERCISES (10 MINUTES)

Stretching by itself is not a warmup. The previous exercises were for that. Don't substitute stretching for them. Warmups start the blood flowing in your muscles. Stretching makes them more flexible. Also, stretch with static movements, not ballistic movements. This allows a better range of motion and reduces the chance of injury.

Hold a stretch for at least 20 seconds, exhaling into the stretch and inhaling out of it.

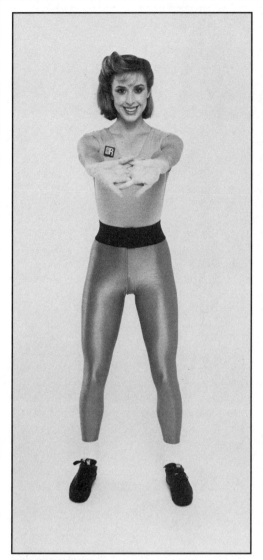 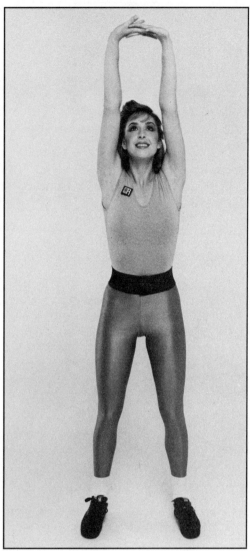

CEILING PRESS

Interlace your fingers, then straighten your arms out in front of you with palms facing out. Hold that for about 20 seconds. Now turn your palms upward above your head as you straighten your arms. Imagine pressing up against the ceiling as you stretch and hold the position.

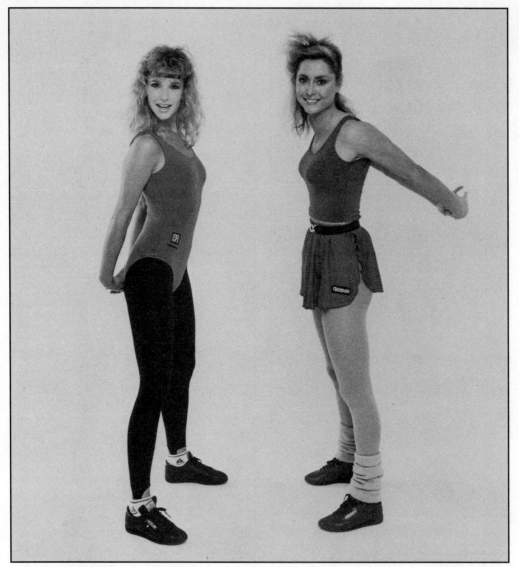

SHOULDER STRETCH
Stand erect with feet shoulder-width apart, and clasp your hands behind your back. Relax your knees and slowly raise your arms as far as you can comfortably reach. Hold for about 20 seconds.

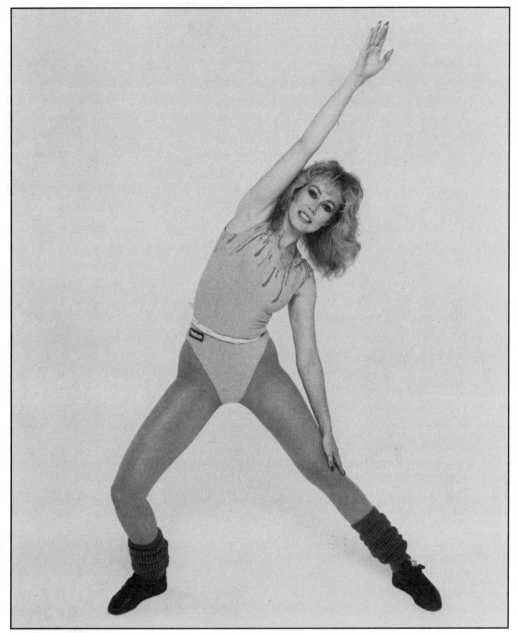

WAIST STRETCH

Stand erect with your feet just beyond shoulder-width apart. Bend your right knee and reach your left hand down the left side of your leg as far as you can. Hold your left hand at this farthest point. Simultaneously, reach your right arm upward past your ear and over your head. Hold for about 20 seconds.

Repeat on the opposite side. Start by bending the left knee and reaching the right hand down the right side, etc.

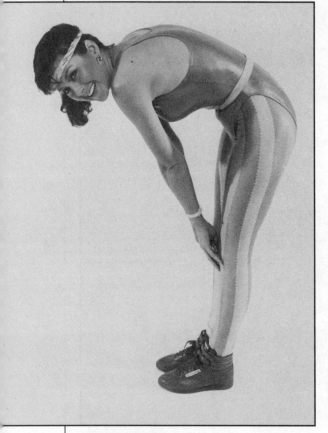 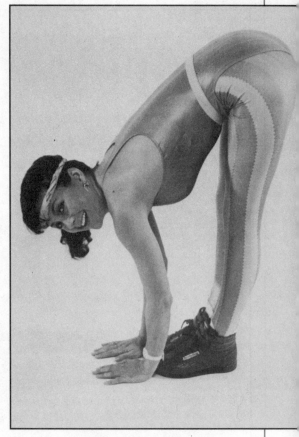

TOE TOUCHES

Stand erect, feet slightly apart and tuck in your abdomen. Curve your head forward, round your back and let the weight of your head pull you down toward the floor as far as you can go. Then roll back up with knees slightly bent. Repeat the movement slowly, with control. Don't fling your body up and down.

Now roll your head and body back down to your farthest point. Bend your knees until your palms can touch the floor. Press the palms flat on the floor and try to straighten the legs without taking your palms off the floor. Don't bounce to get lower.

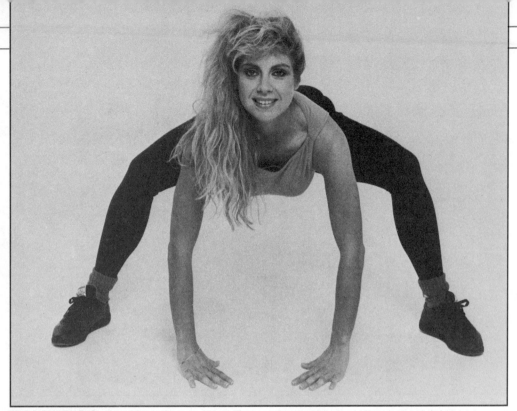

FROG STRETCH

From a standing position with feet just beyond shoulder-width apart, squat down with your feet flat on the floor and toes slightly turned out. Lean forward, bending your knees, and place your hands on the floor for balance. Now lower chest to your farthest point, keeping the hips up, and hold.

   Note: While in the squatting position, check your alignment, as in the detail photo below. Your lower leg is practically straight, with the heel under the knee. Each foot should be flat on the floor.

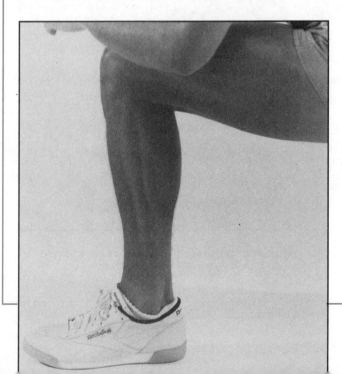

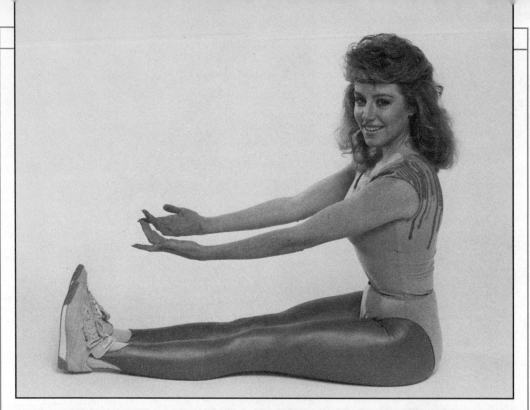

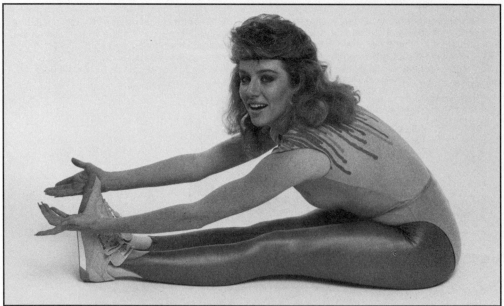

TRUNK FLEXION
Sit up straight, flat on the floor with legs fully extended in front of you with feet flexed, toes pointed up. Without rounding your lower back, lean forward and slowly reach toward your feet.
  Note: Don't lock your knees. Relax them.

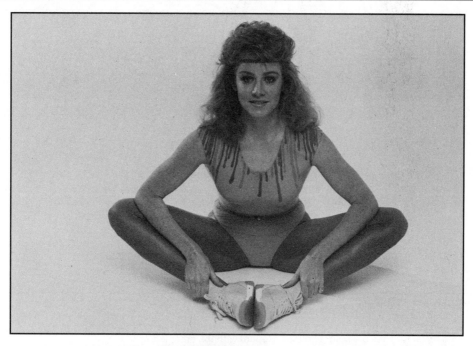

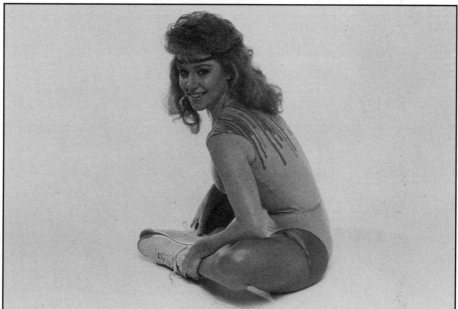

GROIN STRETCH

Sit up straight on the floor and bend your knees, placing the soles of your feet together. Your hands are holding your ankles not your feet. Gently pull your upper body forward with a straight back until you feel a comfortable stretch. Slowly roll back up.

Note: Do this exercise bending forward from your hips. Do not bend or round your back.

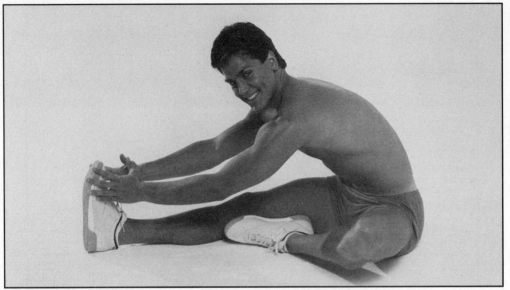

HURDLER STRETCH
Sitting up in the groin-stretch position, straighten the right leg but keep the left knee bent. The right foot should be flexed, but don't lock your knees. Now once again bend forward from the hips, reaching as far as possible before holding. Repeat with the other leg.

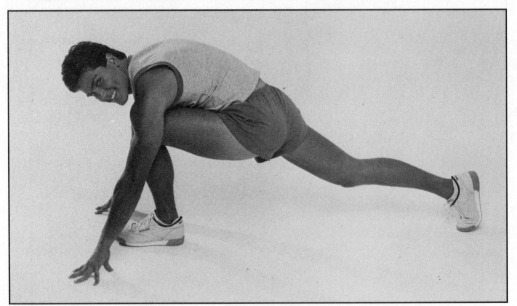

LUNGE
From a kneeling position, move the right leg forward until the knee of the forward leg is directly over your toes. Lean forward until your hands are on the floor on either side of your right leg. Push the left leg far enough behind and straighten your leg without locking the knee. Without changing your position, gently press the front of your hip downward. Repeat with other leg.

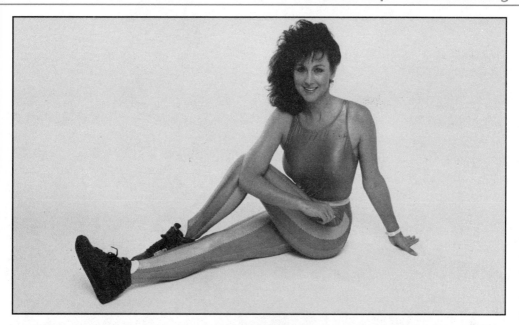

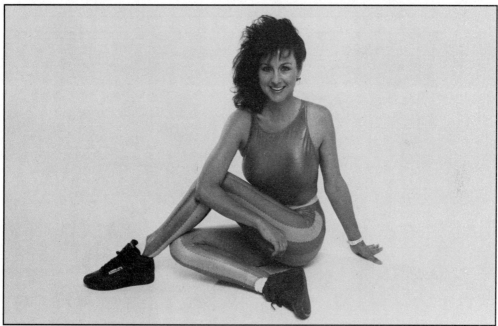

SPINAL TWIST
Sit up straight on the floor with your right leg outstretched in front. Bend your left knee and cross your left foot over to rest next to the outside of your right knee. Now bend your right leg sideways so that the right heel is near your left hip. Bend your right elbow and rest it on the outside of your upper left thigh just above the knee. Slowly press the left hip on the floor. Control this pressure at the same time, looking over your left shoulder. Repeat with other side.

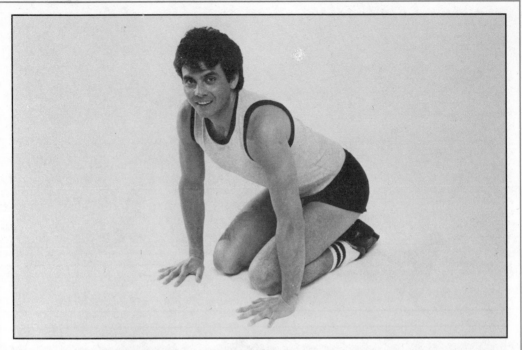

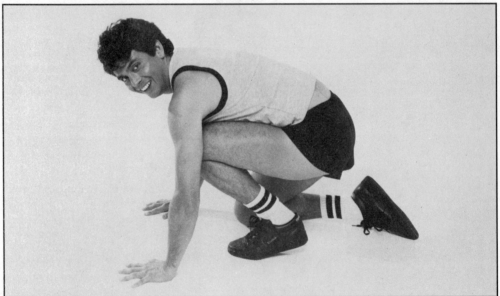

ACHILLES STRETCH
Kneel on the ground with your buttocks resting on your heels. Your feet should not be turned out. Bend your left leg in front. Now bring the toes of your left foot almost even or parallel to your right knee. Place your hands on the floor in front of you. Let the heel of the bent leg come off the ground about a half inch or so. Now lower the heel toward the floor while pushing forward on your thigh—just above the knee—with your chest and shoulders. Repeat with other leg.

COOLDOWN EXERCISES (10 MINUTES)

Cooling down is important because it assists your muscles in pumping blood from your extremities back to the heart. Immediately after the aerobic portion and just before your cooldown exercises, take your pulse to determine whether it is too high, too low or at the target heart rate.

For your cooldown exercises, consider reversing the order of the warmup exercises. In other words, slow down to a jog, then alternate bent knee lifts with side-to-side shuffles. We suggest that you complete your cooldown exercises with at least three to five minutes of stretching exercises too. But remember, before you stretch, take your pulse again to make sure it is less than 100.

Although the warmup, flexibility and cooldown exercises are not new creations, the combination and the order we recommend are unique to a well-balanced MuscleAerobics program.

MUSCLEAEROBICS ON A STATIONARY BICYCLE

A stationary bicycle is one of the most effective and injury-free aerobic aids available. Adding a MuscleAerobics program to a stationary-bicycle workout brings a new dimension to training. This type of exercise is also a super alternative to conventional MuscleAerobics. Those exercises start on page 115. You will benefit and progress from a variety of exercises.

You can do MuscleAerobics on a stationary bicycle at home or in a health club. At home, consider setting it up in front of your television. Watch 30 minutes fly by as you view your favorite program.

Doing MuscleAerobics on a health-club's bicycle may soon make you the center of attention. Everyone will want to know what you're doing and why. It's also a great way to make new friends while staying in shape.

We do MuscleAerobics on a stationary bicycle as an alternate workout. This allows us to use a heavier handweight, rather than increase the intensity level on the bicycle. In fact, when you feel ready for heavier weights, begin by using them on a stationary bicycle. This way your lower body is positioned firmly on the bicycle so you can focus your attention on controlling the arm movements.

Starting Out—Do the same type of warmups and stretches described earlier for conventional MuscleAerobics. They're essential before you get on the bike.

Sit on the bicycle and push down on the right pedal with your foot. You should adjust the seat so that your right leg is straight and the knee slightly bent, as shown in the following photos.

Start pedaling and let the weights swing forward and backward by your side for about a minute. This allows your body to adjust to the bike and weights. Then get a firm, but relaxed, grip on the weights and let them swing up higher, closer to your shoulders.

After you've been on the bike pedaling for about three minutes, your arms should be swinging beyond your shoulders and overhead. At this point you're ready to experiment with the different exercises we've designed. During your bike ride, don't let the weights dangle by your side. Keep them swinging. If you start to fatigue, lower the weights and alternate swinging them at your side.

MUSCLEAEROBICS ON WHEELS

We've created some themes for the exercises. The names mimic common athletic motions to help you remember them better.

Beginners use the same exercises as intermediate and advanced exercisers. Simply start with the minimum number of repetitions and slowly progress as endurance improves.

In the following descriptions, a *set* is a combination of movements or the complete exercise as described. In most cases this will combine movements for both left and right sides. A *rep* or *repetition* is how many times you do a single movement.

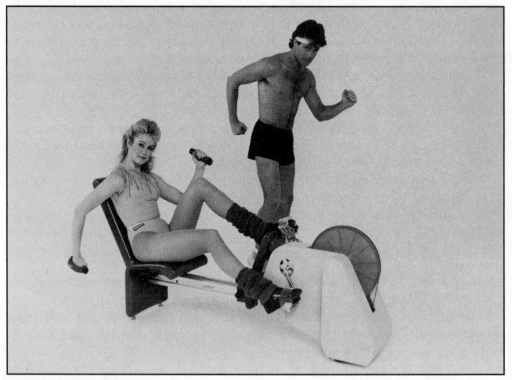

TRIATHLETE RUNNING
Begin with your arms at your side, elbows bent. Alternately pump your arms in front of you for 5 to 10 sets or more.
   Repeat the whole set at least once and you will be ready for the Ironman.

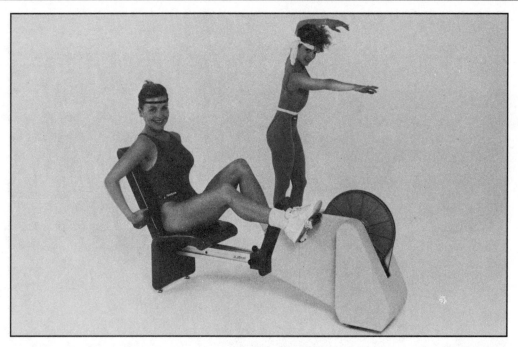

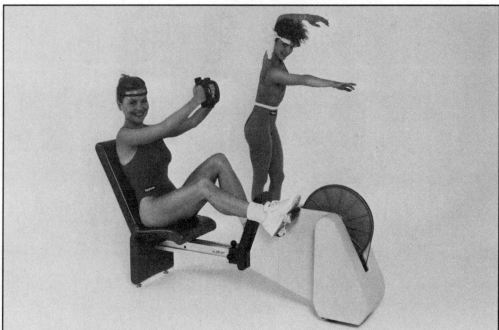

TRIATHLETE SWIMMING
Begin with your arms at your side, elbows bent. Swing your arms forward to eye level, bringing the weights together and return. Keep the momentum going for 5 to 10 sets or more.

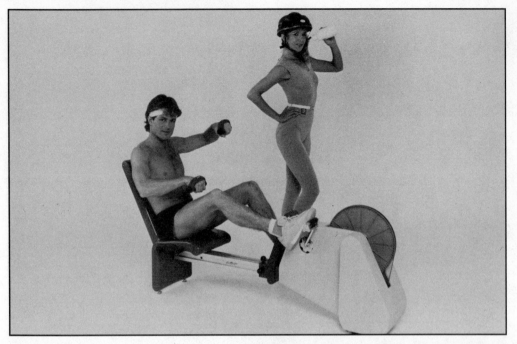

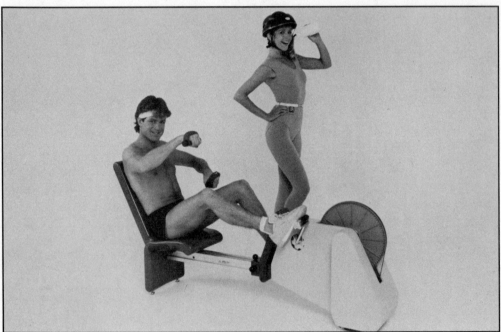

TRIATHLETE BIKING
Bring your arms out directly in front of you and move your arms in a circular fashion, mimicking the motion of your feet pedaling the bike. Maintain this momentum for 5 to 10 sets or more.

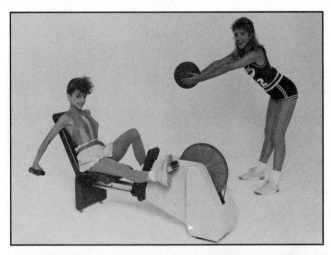

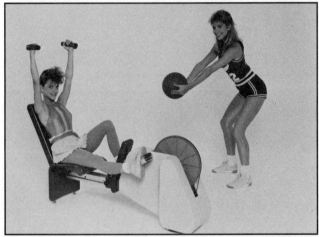

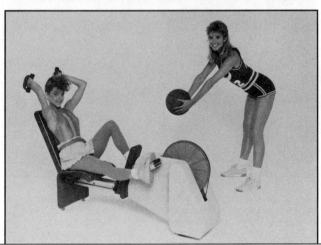

FREE THROW

Swing your arms straight overhead. Hold, then bend and straighten your elbows. Next swing the arms back. The motion you create is: lift-hold-bend-straighten-swing back. Repeat this one set 10 to 20 times or until you make a basket.

Variation: When you swing your arms up, hold them overhead and bend and straighten your elbows for 5 to 10 repetitions.

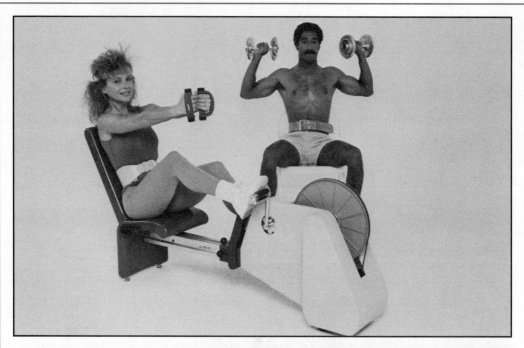

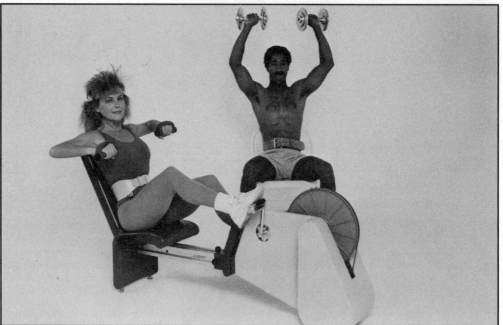

BENCH PRESS
Pump both your arms in front of you so the weights are parallel to each other oriented vertically. When you bring the weights back to a bent elbow position, twist the weights so they are horizontal. (The twist begins when you start to bend the elbows to pull the weights back.) Do 30 to 50 sets.

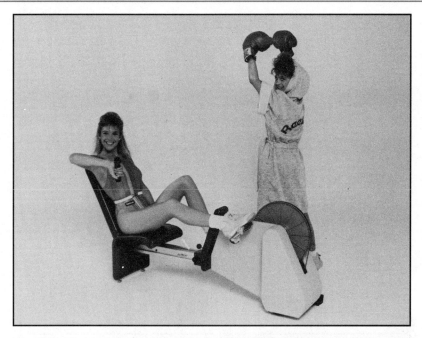

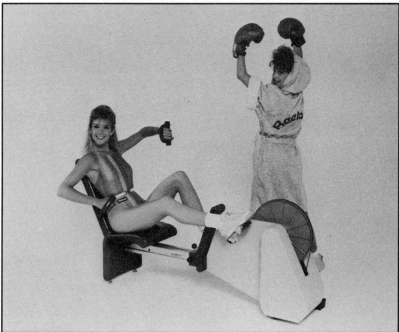

LEFT AND RIGHT HOOK
Hold your weights at your waist. Keeping the elbow bent, raise your right arm out at ear level. Repeat with left side. Alternate your "hooks" for at least 10 to 30 sets or until you really give someone the hook.

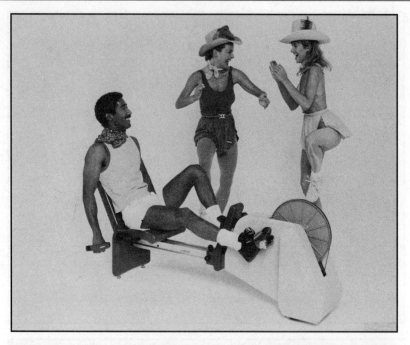

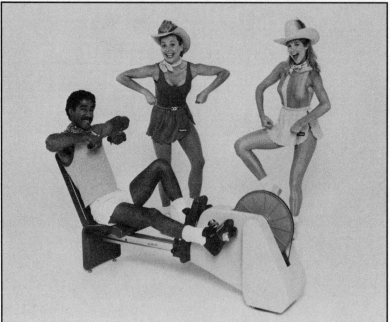

HOE DOWN
Start with your arms straight down on each side of you. Keeping your arms at your side with your weights in a horizontal position, bend your elbows completely in, bringing the weights almost to your armpits. Continue this action until the cows come home or 20 to 50 counts, whichever occurs first.

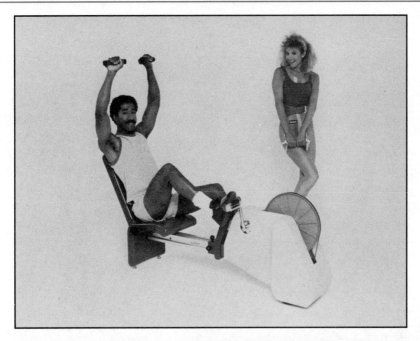

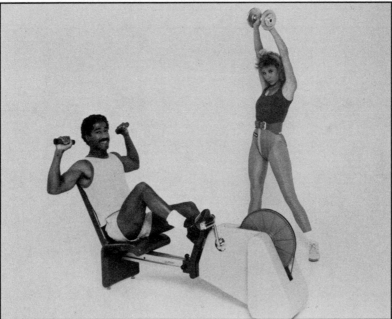

OVERHEAD PRESS
This is a great weightlifting technique for your shoulders and upper back. Pump your arms directly overhead and return them to shoulder level, elbows bent. You're ready for your first bodybuilding contest after 20 to 50 repetitions.
    Variation: Alternate the pumping of your arms.

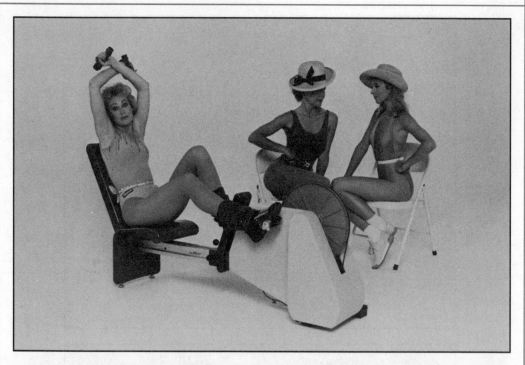

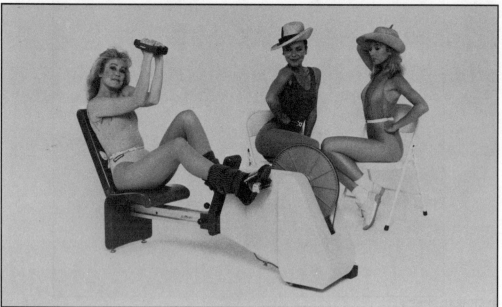

CONVERSATION PIECE
If you thought the other exercises made you conspicuous, this one will really get people talking. Cross your arms behind your head with bent elbows. Uncross them and while keeping your elbows bent, bring them together in front of you at chest level. Keep the folks talking for 10 to 30 sets.

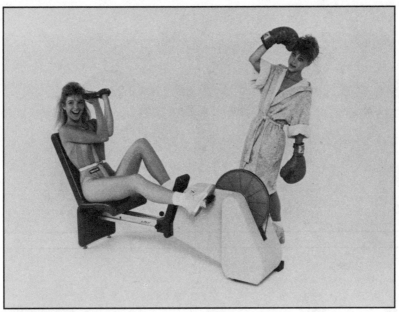

KNOCK YOURSELF OUT
Either fatigue or carelessness will cause you to "knock yourself out" with this one. To give your biceps a good workout, hold your arms directly in front of you with the palms of your hands facing up. Bend and straighten your arms completely. Do 10 to 30 curls before you get knocked out!
    Variation: Alternate your curls.

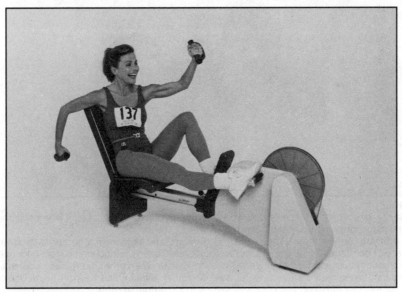

GOING FOR THE FINISH
Starting with both elbows bent at your side, alternate a fast-paced straightening and bending of your arms with a pumping action. Make sure you completely straighten and bend your arms. Sprint for at least a minute or two.

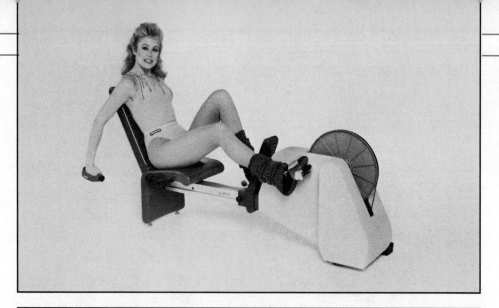

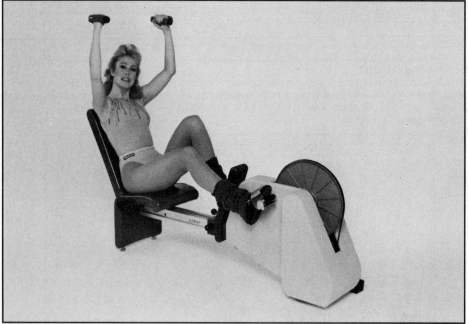

THE SWING

This is a standard move for MuscleAerobics on a stationary bicycle. You used it when starting out. You can also incorporate it into the regimen, as follows:

Starting with your arms at your side, swing them forward and backward together, with controlled movements. But don't turn into a grandfather's clock pendulum by letting momentum take over.

We recommend this movement when you start to fatigue or when other exercises become too difficult. You can swing at three levels: waist level, shoulder level and above your head. Use the swing as your transitional exercise when you switch from routine to routine.

NORDIC SKIING

This routine isn't pictured, but it's similar to The Swing. The only difference is that you alternate the arm swinging. Take off and ski the countryside for about two or three minutes steadily.

THE MUSCLEAEROBICS CHALLENGE

The following exercises are specifically designed for Beginning, Intermediate and Advanced MuscleAerobics Programs. For example, the Beginning MuscleAerobics Program uses constant movements for both the upper and lower body *without* running in place. This helps the beginner get the feel of the weight and motions before combining it with running. However, if you are a beginner who feels ready to jog a bit, do incorporate slow jogging with the movements.

The Intermediate MuscleAerobics Program encourages jogging or "faster" running in conjunction with the arm/handweight movements. The routines are designed to keep your heart pumping at a "middle-of-the-road" intensity level.

The Advanced MuscleAerobics Program achieves the highest intensity. There are nonstop lower- and upper-body moves. Arm movements are mostly overhead. Knees are high. Leg kicks are at waist level, and foot movements are fast. As you become more advanced, feel free to add additional weight. However, make sure that you can still control the extra weight. If the movements become out of control, keep your feet moving at a fast pace, but slow the arm movements. If control is still a problem, consider building strength by using the heavier weights on a stationary bicycle and the lower weights when running in place.

Since we're offering you a "Fitness Menu," feel free to pick and choose *any* of the routines and make them applicable to your fitness level. Your combined MuscleAerobics routines should involve at least 20 minutes, but preferably 30 minutes, of nonstop movements. This time *does not include* your warmup, stretching and cooldown exercises.

Remember to keep the energy flow consistent. Move along steadily without any breaks. To insure proper intensity, select all your exercise routines ahead of time. This way, you won't have to stop and think which one you would like to do next, thereby breaking the flow. Have fun mixing and matching with your favorite upbeat music.

There's no time like the present—so put on some comfortable clothes, clear the floor and let's warmup for the MuscleAerobics challenge!

BEGINNING MUSCLEAEROBICS

The greatest display of sports excellence is clearly the Olympic Games. To make your Beginning MuscleAerobics Program as exciting and goal-oriented as possible, we've created an Olympic theme for each of the exercises.

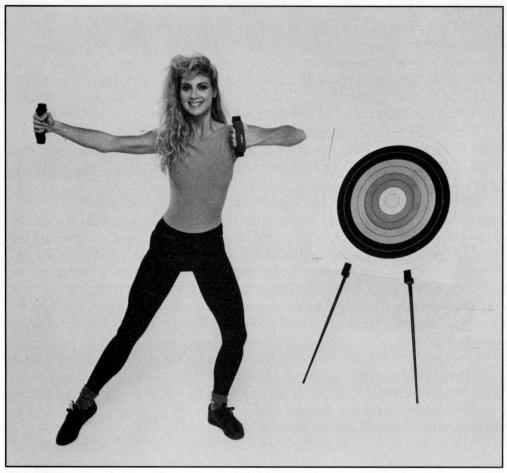

ARCHERY
Extend your left leg out to the side, touching your toe on the floor and letting your right leg bear the weight. At the same time, extend your left arm out to the side, mimicking a pull on your imaginary bow with your right arm. Repeat with other side. That's one set.

Create continuous bow-and-arrow motions and side-to-side foot movements for a minimum of eight sets.

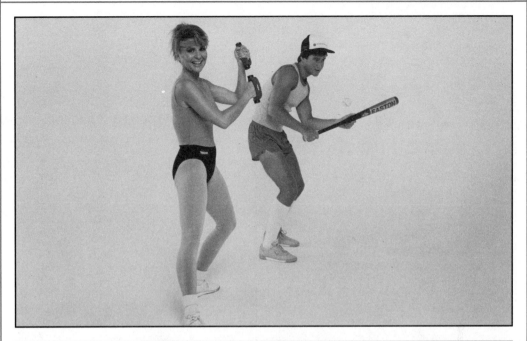

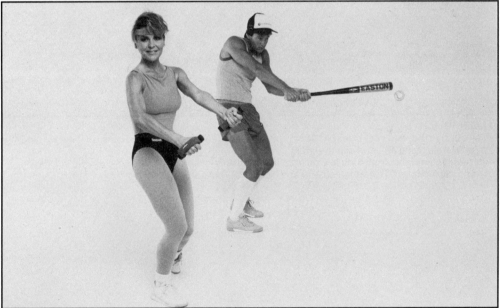

BASEBALL

Step forward with your left leg. Now have your right foot step beside your left while swinging your weights together as if they form an imaginary baseball bat.

Continue the movement by bringing the right leg back and having the left foot step together with the right, while returning the "bat" to your starting position. Do at least 10 swings before switching sides—unless you "strike out" sooner!

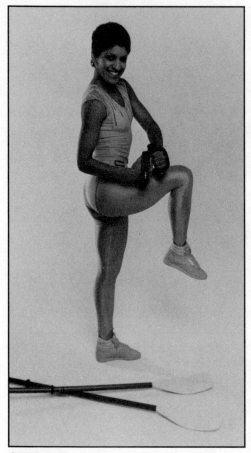 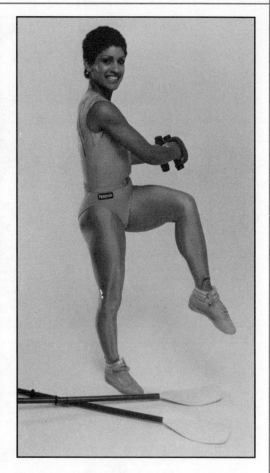

CANOEING

Raise your right knee to your chest while both arms are together. Move the weights on the right side as if you were moving an oar through water.

Alternate the weights from side to side, continuing the movement as if you were rowing in a canoe. Row for a minimum of 10 repetitions, slow and controlled. No tipping over.

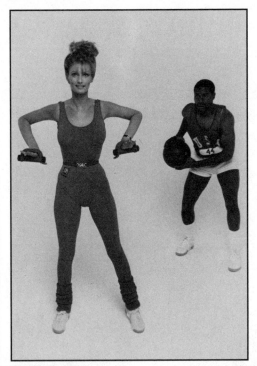 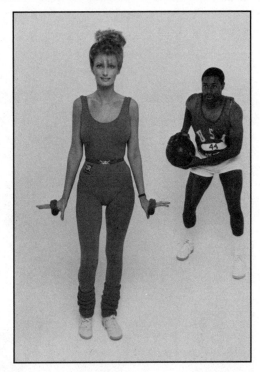

BASKETBALL
Extend the left leg to the side then step with the right to bring legs together. Now extend the right leg to the side, then step together. This is called a *side-to-side shuffle.* Your arms are at your side, and as you shuffle you straighten and bend the elbows vigorously. It's as if you were double-dribbling two basketballs. Dribble the full court or 10 sets.

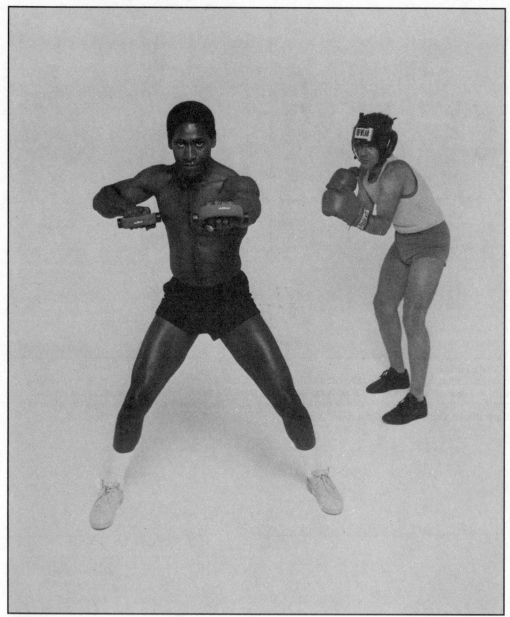

BOXING
Hold arms straight out, slightly below shoulder level but even with your chest. Alternate left and right punches while performing the side-to-side shuffle. Knock out after 40 punches.

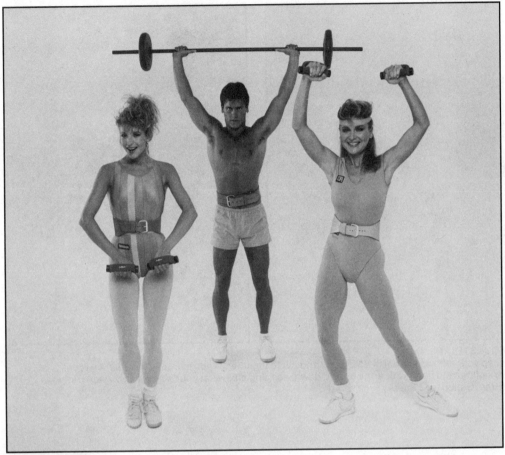

POWERLIFTING
Starting with your weights in front of you at your waist, with one movement bring them directly overhead and then back to your waist while doing the side-to-side shuffle. For beautiful shoulders, lift a minimum of 15 repetitions.

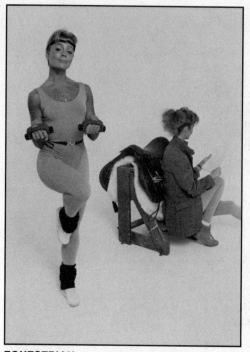 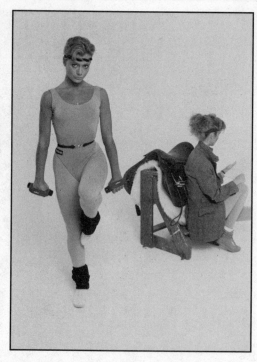

EQUESTRIAN
Keep your elbows in front of your body and close together. While marching around the room, straighten and bend your arms up and down, keeping elbows at your side as if you were riding a horse. Gallop for 15 sets.

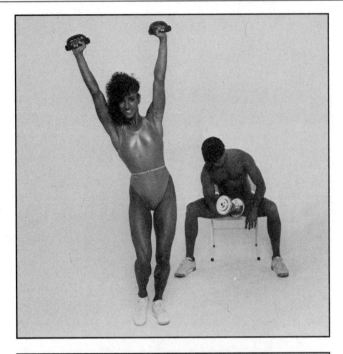

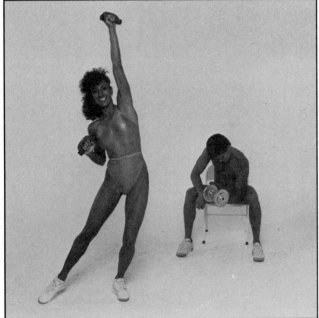

WEIGHTLIFTING
Press the weights directly overhead. Now do the side-to-side shuffle replacing the step with a kick.
Pump the weights up and down overhead accompanying each kick. "Max out" at 20 reps.
  Variation pictured: Alternate left and right pumps of the weights.

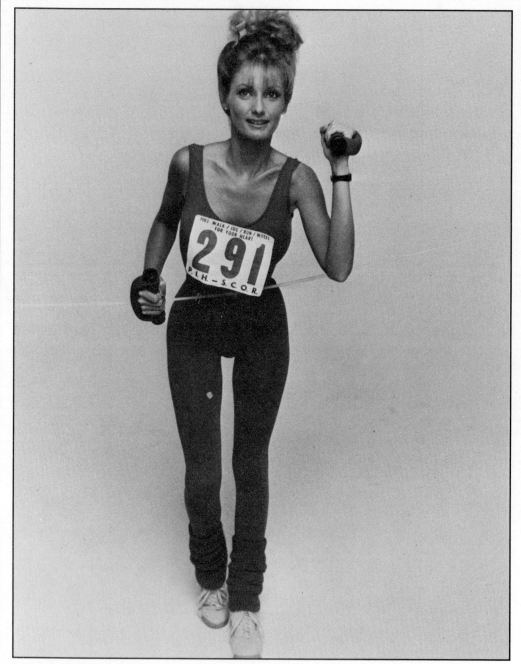

RACEWALKING
Pump your arms vigorously while walking quickly around the room in one direction for approximately one minute. Switch directions for another minute. Walk in circles for two minutes or "until you get there."

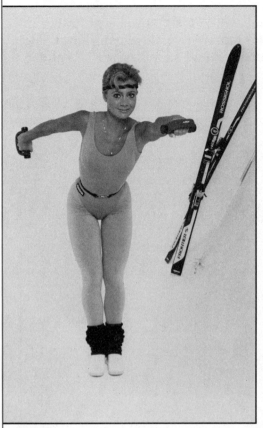 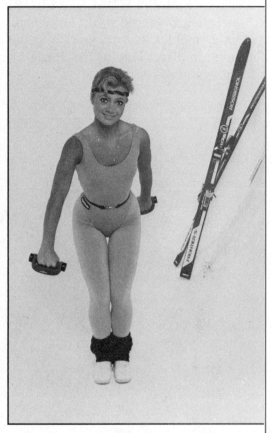

SKIING
With bent knees, create a bouncing-hip action while swinging the left arm forward and right arm back. Repeat with other arm. Stop at 30 sets or until frostbitten.

INTERMEDIATE MUSCLEAEROBICS

Having advanced to the intermediate level, you are now a step further in MuscleAerobics. This program incorporates more active movements, including running in place. Due to the upbeat nature of these exercises, we've entitled this program *Movin' in Style*.

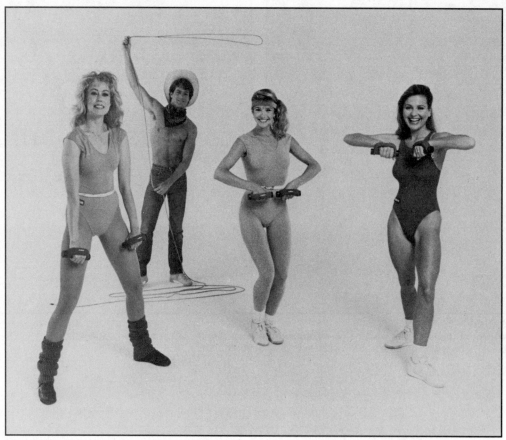

GOING TO THE RODEO

Shuffle and step, moving from one end of the room to the other, keeping your weights together and continuously moving them up to the chest and down to the waist, bending the elbows completely. Your arm motion should mimic a washerwoman or rodeo rider. Take your pick.

The whole routine is continuous. Depending on the size of the room, you'll either circle the room or shuffle from one end to the other. Continue the steps for at least two minutes before moving to your next routine. Be sure to yell *yahoo!* during your shuffling around the corral.

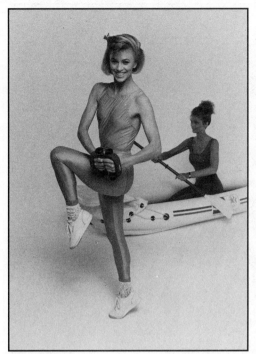 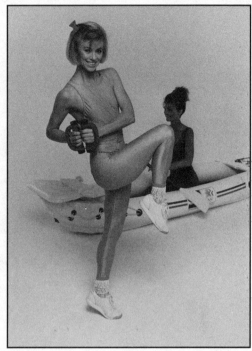

KAYAKING
Hop on one leg while bending and lifting the opposite knee slightly above waist level. Keeping the weights together, move your imaginary oar past the raised knee. Alternate from leg to leg. Continue down the rapids for 40 sets.

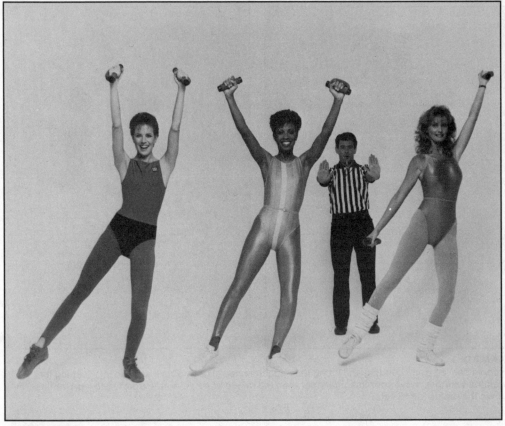

THE REFEREE

Alternate side-to-side kicks maintaining momentum while bringing both arms straight up for two counts. Then form a V-shape with your straight arms for two counts.

Next, hop once on your right foot and kick the left leg out to the side while the left arm is straight up and the right arm is straight down. Now hop on the left foot and kick the right leg out to the side while your right arm is straight up and the left arm is straight down. Caution: After 15 sets you'll be ready to sit on the sidelines.

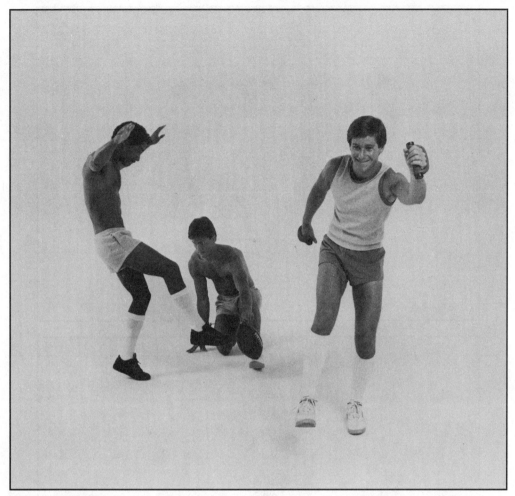

TOUCH FOOTBALL
Alternate kicking left and right legs in front and hopping on the opposite leg as you alternate swings of your left and right arms high in front of you. Keep your arms tight but elbows relaxed. Touchdown is after 40 reps.

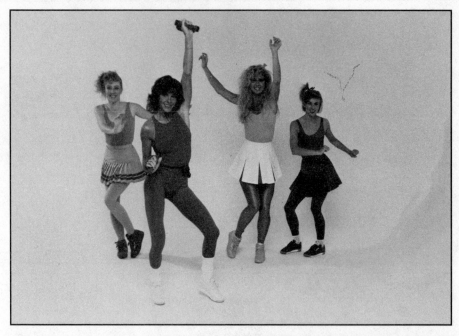

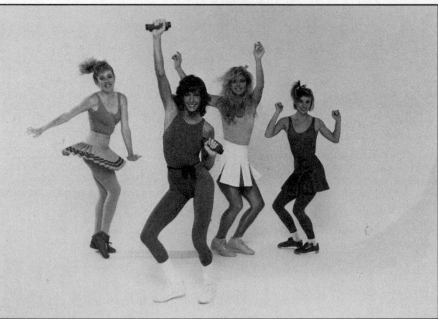

TWIST AND SHOUT
Feet are shoulder-width apart. Hop and twist left to right while alternating the pumping of your arms overhead. Make sure when you pump the weights that you bring your elbow down to your waist while the opposite arm is straight overhead. We've supplied the twist. Now supply the shout part if you like.
  Variation: Twist and hop two counts on the left side, then two counts on the right side.

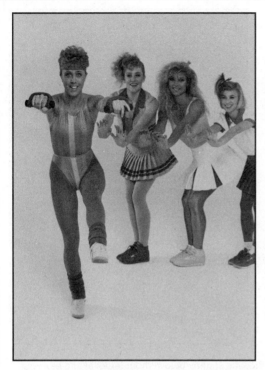

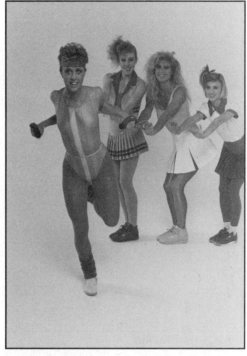

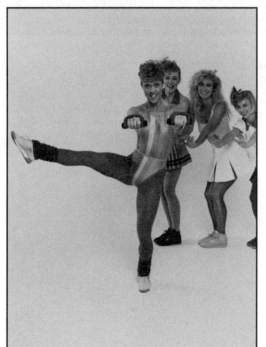

PUSH 'EM BACK

Starting with your left foot, run forward three counts then kick with your right leg on the fourth count. Now step backward with your right foot and run for three counts. Kick your left foot forward on the fourth count. Continue the up-and-back movements while pushing your arms in front to the beat. The beat is *Up-2-3-Kick; Back-2-3-Kick.*

Variation: Move to the right side starting with your right foot. On the third count, turn and face the left side. Then kick your left leg on the fourth count. Step down on that left foot and continue the moves to the left side. Repeat the whole set. Send the team to victory with 10 sets for each variation.

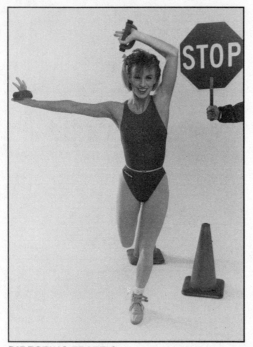
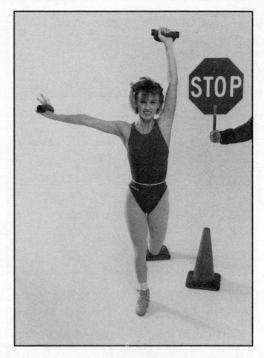

DIRECTING TRAFFIC
While running in place, extend your left arm out to the side slightly below shoulder level and flex your hand. Raise the right arm overhead with the elbow close to your ear. Let the weight point down behind your back. Now extend the arm completely and bend it back completely. Keep the elbow close to the ear and don't move it forward or backward. Perform at least eight repetitions before switching arms to do the next set. No time for tickets during traffic.

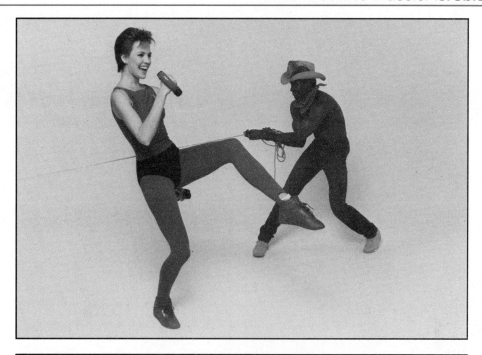

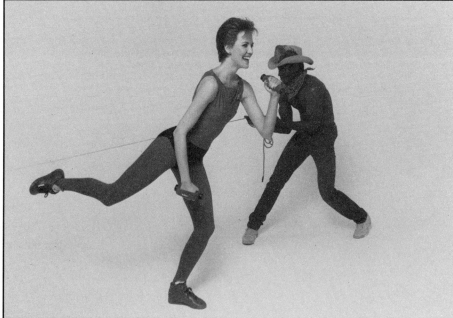

RIDE THE WILD STALLION
Hop back on your right leg, bending the knee while the front left leg is bent and raised close to your chest. Alternate bending and straightening your elbow as you rock forward and backward. Rock at least eight times on each side before switching sides; then dismount.

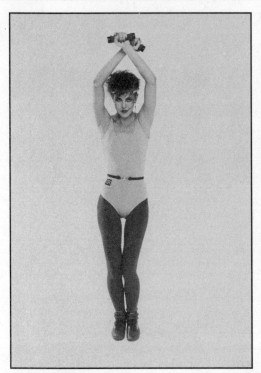 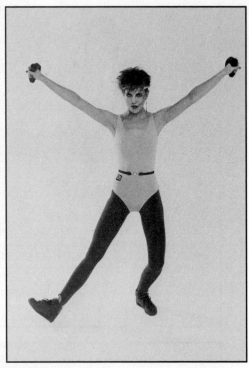

BORN TO BE WILD
Hop once with feet together and cross your arms overhead in front of your face. Hop again, letting your right leg bear the weight, and kick your left leg out to the side, letting your heel touch the ground. While all of this is happening, your arms are overhead and outstretched.

Now hop in the center with your feet together and arms crossed overhead. Finish the move by kicking with your right leg. Perform for 30 counts or until you're arrested.

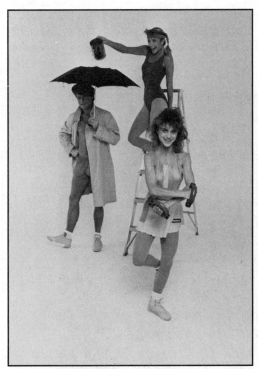 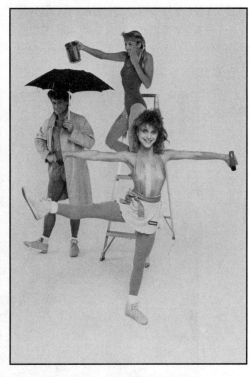

SINGIN' IN THE RAIN
Start with your arms crossed down in front of you. Hop on your right leg while kicking your left leg out to the side. At the same time, uncross your arms and swing them out on either side.

Now hop on your left leg and kick out your right leg to the side. Continue crossing and uncrossing your arms as you kick your legs out. Dance until soaked or you finish 20 sets, whichever comes first.

ADVANCED MUSCLEAEROBICS

You're ready for the big time. It's all uphill from here. After just one workout, you'll understand why our title for this series of exercises is *Sizzlin' Hot*.

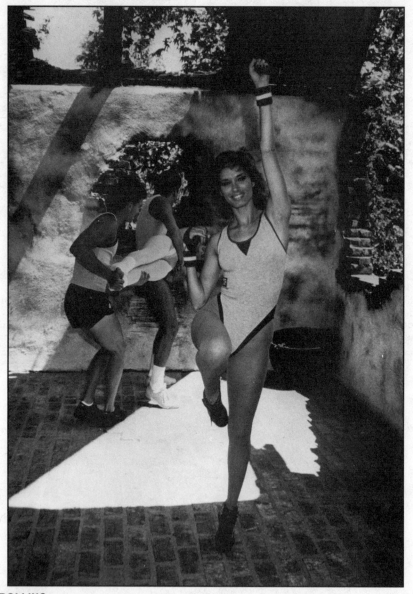

STEAM ROLLING
Alternate high left and right knee lifts with alternating left and right pumps of your arms overhead. Try this for 50 counts and steam will be in great supply.

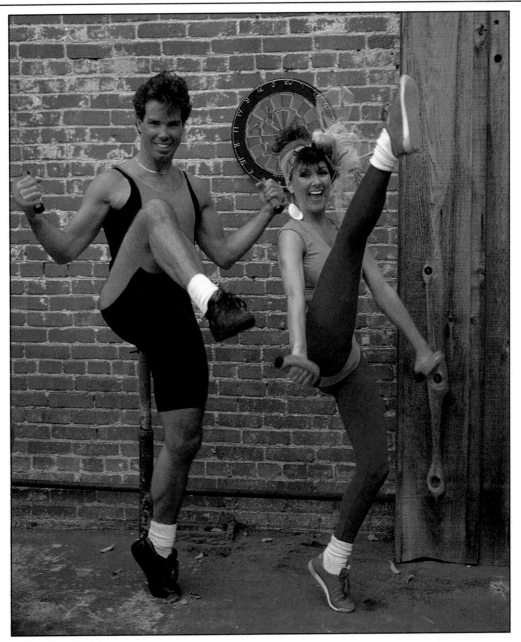

ON TARGET

Those with a little dance fever in them will enjoy this "can-can" exercise. Your arms will be moving up and down with each kick. The leg does not have to be high. Some people are more flexible than others, so pace yourself.

Alternate from leg to leg and make sure you bring the foot through the full range of motion. In other words, don't continue hopping on the ball of your foot. Once you get the hang of this you'll hit the bull's eye. . .let's say after 20 sets.

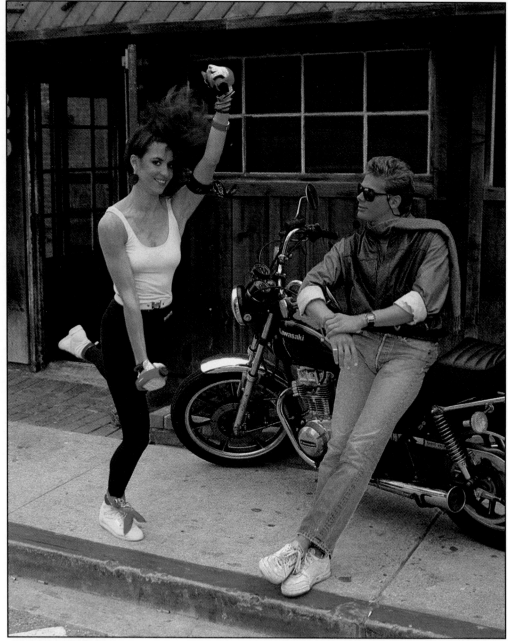

ROUGH AND READY

In this exercise you won't know whether you're coming or going. Lean forward and alternately kick left and right legs behind you for four counts, keeping your knees slightly bent. At the same time, you are alternately swinging your left and right arms in front up and down. As shown on the next page, then alternate kicking your legs in front of you for four counts while pumping your arms directly overhead. You'll be ready for Rocky after 20 sets.

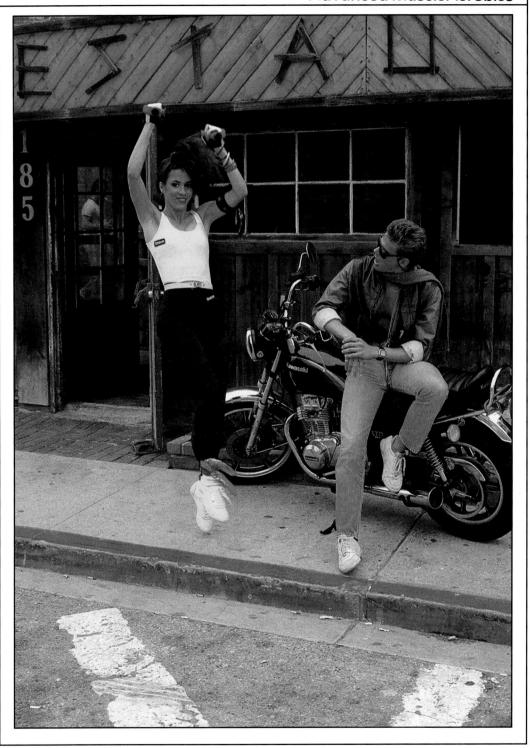

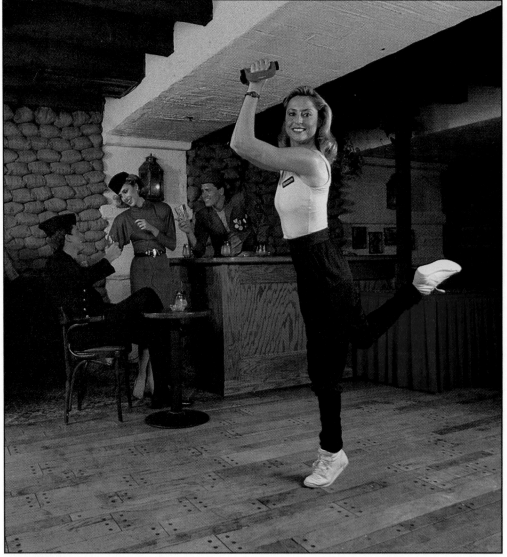

THE TORCH

This exercise may seem relatively easy, but look out. Do it for a while and you'll understand how we named it.

While running in place, bring your arms up and bend your elbows at chest level. Press your elbows together, press your weights together and lift and lower your arms. Burn out after 40 lifts.

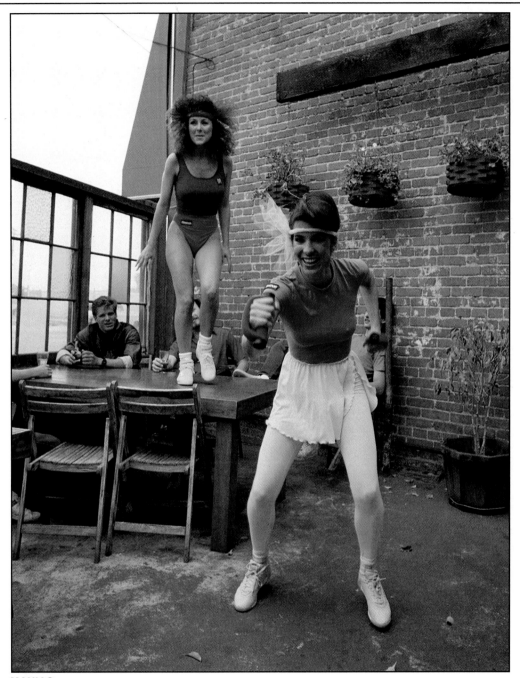

MANIAC
Inspired by the great dancing of the film *FlashDance,* this movement requires a rapid stomping from foot to foot while vigorously pumping your arms as if you were sprinting for the finish line. Legs are positioned just beyond hip-width. If you look like a dancer after 40 counts, be pleased.

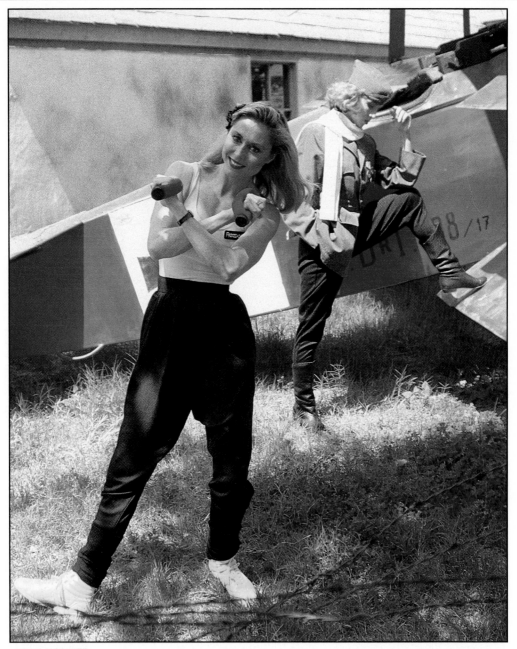

STARFIGHTER

Hop on your right foot while bending the left knee at the same time. Then hop on your left foot and bend the right knee. As you hop from side to side, your arms are directly overhead. Bending your elbows, cross your arms behind your head for two counts. Then bring the arms at chest level and cross them in front for two counts. Alternate your crossing from overhead to chest level. Look out galaxy, here you come! You are sure to feel cosmic after 40 to 50 counts.

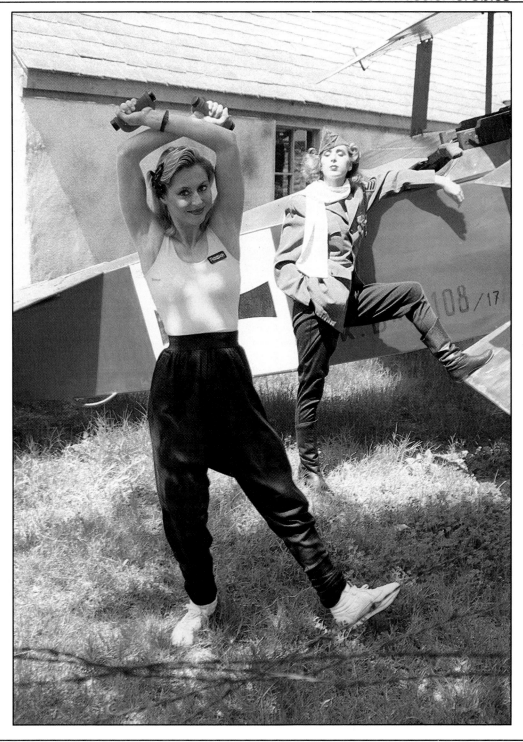

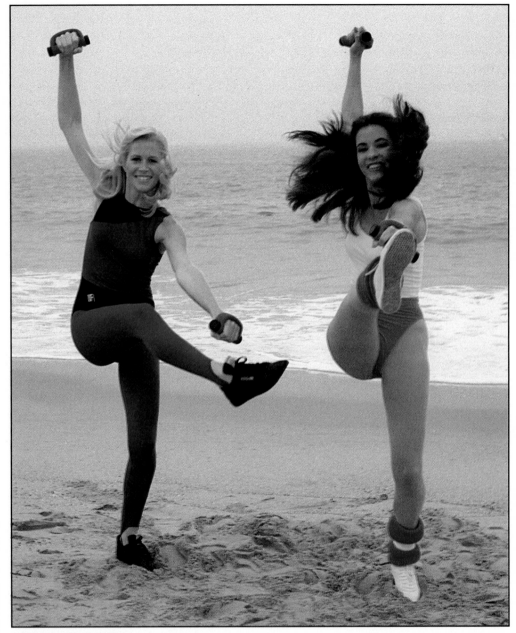

RIDE THE WILD SURF

Let's try bodysurfing, MuscleAerobics style. Hop on your right foot while lifting and turning out your left knee. Create a swimming motion so your right arm comes around and touches your left foot as it is raised.

Bring the other arm around in a swimming stroke, while hopping on your left foot. At the same time, raise and turn out the right knee and touch the right foot. Alternate from leg to leg and go for a long ride. Wipe out after 20 sets.

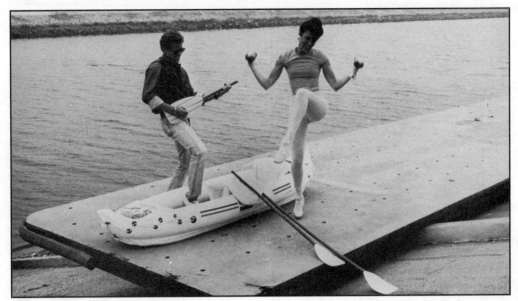

ROCK AND ROW
While hopping on your left foot, raise the right knee to your chest. Hop and lift the knee twice to the right while moving your arms straight up and down with the rhythm. Repeat this move on the left side. This ought to send you more than "merrily down the stream," especially after 40 sets.

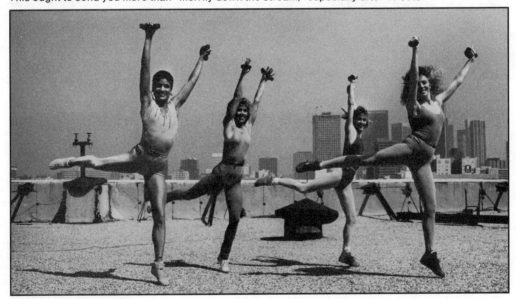

REACH FOR THE STARS
Swing both arms to the right while hopping on your right foot and kicking to the side with your left leg. Position your body to face the right side. Repeat the move on the left side, then alternate from side to side. You'll be light years ahead of the rest after 40 to 50 counts.

   Variation: Kick twice while swinging on the right side. Then kick twice swinging on the left side and repeat.

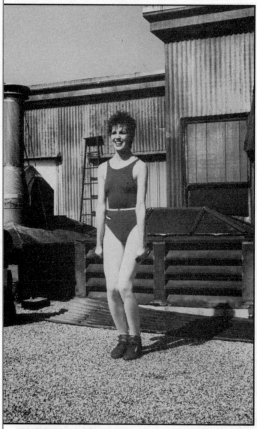 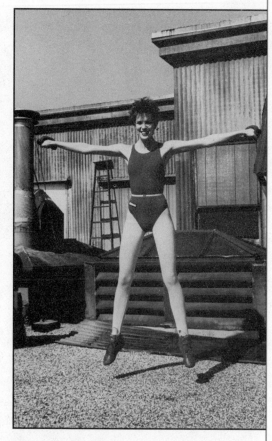

THE FURNACE

There's no better name for this fat-burning, jumping-jacks exercise. If your music is too fast, you might lose control, so use an intermediate beat. As you do the jumping-jack, make sure your knees are always bent. Tighten the arms to get maximum benefit. Your fire will be stoked after 100 counts.

CHAPTER SEVEN

Available Weights

Because light handweights are the important tools of MuscleAerobics, we think it is a "weighty" topic. Fortunately, the growing popularity of upper-body conditioning has motivated sporting-equipment manufacturers to research and develop new and improved designs. The result is a growing selection of weights, allowing you to find just the right one.

Visit a local sporting-goods store and explore what's available in light handweights. Use the opportunity to feel the different types available. Your comfort and ability to use the weights are critical to successful MuscleAerobics.

EXPERT ADVICE

To help you further, we've contacted numerous manufacturers of light handweights and have summarized their products and specifications. It's important to invest some time in selecting the equipment. The following advice and tips from physical therapists and exercise physiologists will make your decision more informed.

More Is Not Better—David Pevsner, registered physical therapist and Associate Director of the JMP Center for Sports Medicine and Fitness in Southern California, claims that the Center sees "a lot of shoulder problems that come from the use of arm weights by people who aren't strong enough or who don't use them in a controlled fashion."

Many people fall victim to the "more-is-better syndrome." It's easy to think that a one-pound weight is much too light when holding it in your hand. So why not use three-pound weights? Even if you are accustomed to lifting weights, aerobic weights deal with a different type of stress—constant movement. As a result, you can't compare aerobic weights with heavier weights if the exercises and movements are different.

In this case, more is not better. Starting with a one-pound weight is much easier on your joints. And it will still give you MuscleAerobic benefits.

Grip Considerations—Jacqueline Ross, a physical therapist in New York City with an expertise in sports medicine, cautions against overgripping the handweights. She stresses a relaxed grip when you do MuscleAerobics. When you grip the weight tightly, Ross says that you create an *isometric tension*. This results in too much stress in neck and shoulder muscles.

Many times, especially during an aerobics class, you may find yourself overgripping the weight in an effort to keep up with the movements. You may also be worried that if you loosen your grip, you might lose the weight and possibly knock someone in the head. Our advice is to either loosen the grip or slow the pace.

Ross recommends the following test when trying out handweights: Perform at least 10 repetitions of an isolated movement. For example, hold the weight in your hand and swing your arms forward and backward. If your arm starts to shake and you tend to overgrip, the weight is too heavy.

Safety Considerations—Linda Shelton, an exercise physiologist, stresses the importance of safety during aerobic exercise. She advises against any movements that overstress the shoulder. In particular, she points out that you should not sweep large circles with your arms, especially when using handweights. These ''arm circles'' done incorrectly stress the shoulder even if you don't use weights!

As an added precaution, Shelton advises against using weights heavier than 2-1/2 pounds each. Last but not least, she emphasizes proper breathing, especially when using weights.

Summary—There are five key points to remember:

1) Choose a weight that fits and feels comfortable.
2) Never overgrip the weight.
3) Always maintain control of your movements.
4) Don't increase the amount of weight until you're ready.
5) Keep your body relaxed when exercising.

WHAT'S AVAILABLE

Now you're ready for our rundown of popular weights that are available for MuscleAerobics. The chart on the following page and the accompanying photos cover readily available products.

Aerobic Weights Summary

	Can Add/Subtract Weight	Handweight	Wristweight	Handwrap	Aid Against Overgripping	Balanced Weight Placement	Various Weight Increments	Available Locally	Available Mail Order	WEIGHT AMOUNTS AVAILABLE							Other Features
										1/2 lb.	1 lb.	2 lbs.	3 lbs.	4 lbs.	5 lbs.	6 lbs. or more	
AMF Heavyhands	X	X				X	X	X				X	X	X	X		Hand strap
Fit Stik		X	X			X	X	X	X		X	X	X	X			Instr. manual
The Band				X	X	X	X	X	X		X	X	X	X			Instr. manual
The Softbell		X	X			X		X	X							X	Soft, padded dumbbell
Wonder Weights		X	X	X		X	X	X	X			X	X				Fashion colors
Elmer's Weights		X		X		X	X	X				X	X				Five colors
Soft Weights		X				X	X	X	X	X		X					Adjustable strap
Gymjazz	X	X			X		X	X	X	X							Waterproof
Weider Beauti-Bells		X			X	X		X	X						X	X	Rubbercoated; colors
Weider Wrist Weights			X			X	X	X	X		X						Fashion colors
Slim-Ez		X	X						X								Variable weight
Divajex (Denise Austin)		X		X			X		X	X							Fits on back of hand
Fitness Weight Gloves	X	X					X	X	X								Small, med., and lg.
Xerweight		X						X	X		X	X	X	X	X	X	Std. dumbbell

149

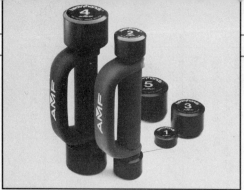

AMF Heavyhands are pictured in use throughout this book. They are cushioned for comfort, easy gripping and let you add or subtract balanced weight. Heavyhands are widely available at sporting-goods and department stores.

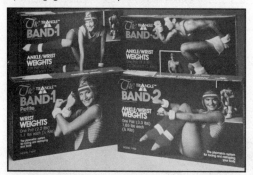

The Triangle Band is a wristweight that easily wraps around the wrist, so there's nothing to hold. Your hands can't overgrip. The Band is sold at sporting-goods stores.

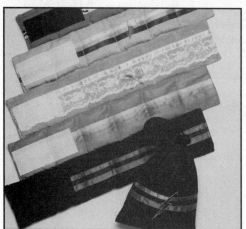

Wonder Weights are "designer-workout" weights, color-coordinated to match the latest leotards and sportswear fashions. They are available by mail order only. For more information, write Wonder Concepts, Inc., 7075 Redwood Boulevard, Suite H, Novato, CA 94947. Or, call 415-898-1816.

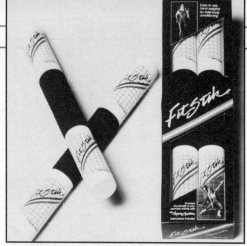

Fit Stiks are baton-shaped and constructed for high-repetition aerobic movements. Fit Stiks are available at sporting-goods and department stores. For additional information, write Aspen Fitness Products, PO Box 4188, Aspen, CO 81612. Or, call 303-920-1543.

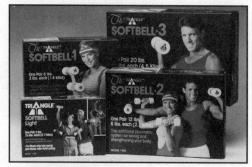

The Triangle Softbell is a soft-cushioned dumbbell. It won't damage floors if dropped. Use the lightest size (1.5 pounds) for a MuscleAerobics program.

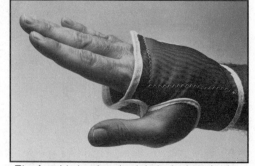

The Aerobic is a handweight is designed to be used while walking, jogging or performing aerobic-conditioning exercises. It's more like a glove than a wristweight. For additional information, call toll-free 800-858-4568.

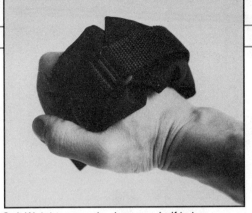

Soft Weights come in sizes one-half to two pounds each. The weight is balanced in one location and can be placed on top of the hand or in the palm. For more information on where to purchase Soft Weights write M. L. Rand Corporation, 3131 Western Avenue, Suite 301 Seattle, WA 98121. Or, call 206-282-3031.

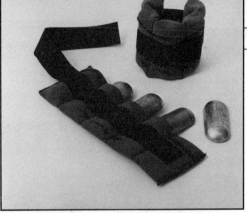

Gymjazz weights are in neoprene cuffs with five chambers that hold removable one-pound and half-pound epoxy-coated weights. They are available in retail and fitness centers nationwide or by mail order: Gymjazz, 8157 Lankershim Blvd., Suite 103, No. Hollywood, CA 91605. Or, call 818-767-7151.

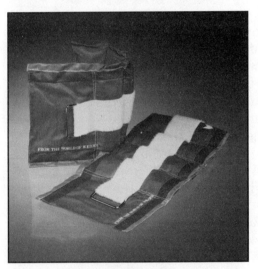

Weider Wrist Weights are available in three- and five-pound sizes. Weider products are available by mail order only. Write Weider Health and Fitness, 21100 Erwin Street, Department MA-1, Woodland Hills, CA 91367. Or call 1-800-423-5713; in California call 1-800-382-3399.

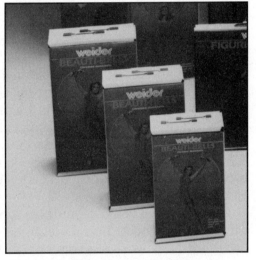

Weider Beauti-Bells are rubber-coated and come in 3-, 5-, 8- and 10-pound pairs. In addition, Weider Products offer chrome dumbbells in a variety of sizes and colors. Available by mail order only. Write Weider Health and Fitness, 21100 Erwin Street, Department MA-1, Woodland Hills, CA 91367. Or call 1-800-423-5713; in California call 1-800-382-3399.

Summary—Because aerobic handweights is a growing area, many sporting-goods manufacturers are developing such weights. Keeping in mind the hand-weight tips you just read about, visit sporting-goods and department stores and ask about their light-, hand- or wristweights. Compare prices, sizes, fit and comfort. Determine which ones best meet your MuscleAerobics needs.

CHAPTER EIGHT

Muscle-Aerobics Case Studies

One day we subtly introduced the concepts of MuscleAerobics in a conventional aerobics class. We *never* suggested that anyone buy weights. As a matter of fact, we never said one word about weights. To our surprise, in a matter of months, about 50% of the class started using light handweights. At the end of one year, almost 75% of a class of approximately 50 people participated in MuscleAerobics *without* our mentioning a thing!

MuscleAerobics is so interesting and versatile that it almost sells itself. In fact, finding people to participate in the case studies of this chapter was easy. The people we selected had already seen us using light handweights in an aerobics class and on a stationary bicycle. They were eager to learn more without any prompting from us.

For our nonscientific, yet thoroughly documented research, we chose two particular individuals that represented opposite sides of the fitness coin. The one thing these two had in common, however, was the fact that MuscleAerobics was a first-time experience for both of them.

We provided them with light handweights and instructed them to monitor their body weight and heart rates. In addition, we asked them to monitor their recovery rates. If you recall in chapter 3, we stated that while exercising, the goal is to continue activity at your target heart rate (THR) for a minimum of 20 minutes.

Once exercise activity is complete, it is just as important that your heart return to normal. The time this takes is called your *recovery rate*. The more physically fit you are, the faster your heart recovers. Ideally, you want your heart to "recover" to 100 beats per minute within two minutes after you cease exercising.

We instructed our case studies to determine how long it took to get their heart rate to 100 beats immediately after they stopped their particular MuscleAerobics program.

They were also instructed to choose either an aerobics-class setting or stationary bicycle and to stick with the program for a specified time span.

Both participants selected the stationary bicycle, which seemed to fit their fitness regime. The stationary bicycle offers various intensity levels rated from 1 to 10 on the machine, signifying degrees of difficulty. A "random" ride creates the illusion of going up and down hills. An "interval" ride refers to a particular time allowing for warmup, training cycle and cooldown. A "manual" ride keeps the intensity level constant throughout the whole ride. Both individuals used all three features during their MuscleAerobics program.

CASE STUDY #1: BRIAN BRASE

Brian Brase, age 26, is a track-and-field coach from California State University, Northridge campus. He agreed to be involved in an eight-week MuscleAerobics study to supplement his present fitness regime.

Prior to the study, Brian's primary daily fitness activities were running and some form of strength training. During the study, Brian averaged from three to five MuscleAerobic workouts per week on the stationary bicycle as a supplement to his regular fitness activities. He started out using two-pound handweights at the beginning of the study. Within three weeks he moved up to five-pound handweights. He devised various movement patterns, which he referred to as MuscleAerobic "medleys." His medleys dealt with movement, weights and bicycle-intensity combinations.

For our study, Brian usually began his ride with simulated hill riding at Random Level 7 for approximately 25 minutes. He concluded it with an Interval Level 7 ride for 12 minutes.

Heart Rates—Before the study, we had Brian ride on the stationary bicycle without using handweights to determine how long it took him to reach his target heart rate. It took him almost 15 minutes to get to his target rate. His recovery at the conclusion of a 45-minute ride was 4 minutes.

Brian experimented with different intensity levels, usually Random Levels 5 to 7, to determine whether they had an affect on his workload. Considering his advanced fitness level, he concluded that his hill riding at Random Level 7 was the intensity he needed for his body to be effectively stressed.

Shortly after he began the study, he was able to reach his target rate within 6 minutes when using light handweights. At the end of his ride, his recovery time dropped to approximately 3 minutes.

Week Two—He then performed a special series of MuscleAerobic medleys that enabled him to get to his target rate faster. The higher he lifted the weights, the faster he achieved his target heart rate. In two weeks' time, he was able to reach his target rate within 5 minutes! That was 10 minutes faster than without weights! He loved getting a better workout in less time.

Weeks Three and Four—By the third week, Brian decreased his intensity riding to Random Level 5 and increased the handweights to 5 pounds. This extra weight took time to get used to, so he restricted his movements to waist height.

He reached his target rate within 4 minutes and his recovery time dropped again, this time to approximately 2 minutes.

In the fourth week, he altered his medleys and reached his target rate within 3 minutes and recovered in 1-1/2 minutes!

Weeks Seven and Eight—When he returned to his two-pound weights by the seventh week, he stated that "The two pounders felt very light as a result of work with five pounders. The five pounders have a strength-training effect as well as adding to my cardiovascular conditioning." He had worked his way to five-pound handweights and decided to stay there.

At the conclusion of the study, on the eighth week, Brian remained at Random Level 7 using five-pound weights. The average time it took to get to his target rate was approximately three minutes. His recovery rate was approximately two minutes. Although his body weight decreased only three pounds—he was in fine shape from the start—he showed a marked improvement in endurance. When asked if he noticed any significant changes, he indicated he felt he got an "intense upper body and cardiovascular workout . . . and my shoulders got bigger as a *direct* result of MuscleAerobics, particularly with the five-pound weights."

Overall, Brian wants to continue on a MuscleAerobics program because he said it allowed for a "much higher quality workout."

Conclusion—We must add that we do not recommend the rapid weight progression Brian adopted. While a MuscleAerobics program allows you to progress to five-pound handweights eventually, it should be a slow progression.

Brian is a perfect example of how MuscleAerobics can continue to benefit the highly trained athlete. One of the major problems for the so-called "superfit" is time. We all want to gain greater endurance, but that also usually means more time. The beauty of a MuscleAerobics program is the ability to increase cardiovascular conditioning, receive a quality workout and get even greater muscular endurance in less time than other plans require.

CASE STUDY #2: CRAIG MENDEL

Such was the case of our next "guinea pig," Craig Mendel, age 25. Craig had an athletic physique, so he wasn't what we would classify as a beginner to fitness. But he was not actively involved in a regular cardiovascular program. His regular fitness routine consisted of karate classes and weight training three times a week, and volleyball and floor hockey once a week.

Although Craig was heavily involved in the family's printing business, he was able to commit to a three-days-a-week program on a stationary bicycle. He remained as a case study for approximately eight weeks, supplementing his regular fitness routine with MuscleAerobics.

We thought we would have a problem keeping Craig involved in the study because he had no desire to participate in aerobic classes and considered the stationary bicycle a boring alternative.

Heart Rates—The first day of the study proved taxing for Craig as our first test was to determine how long it would take to get to his target heart rate while riding the stationary bike without handweights.

After 15 minutes he finally reached his training rate, riding at Random Level 6. Once he reached his target rate, we remember him shouting "How much longer do I have to stay on?" We were able to convince him to remain on the stationary bike for only five additional minutes.

Progress—The next time, we presented him with a one-pound pair of handweights and suggested a few MuscleAerobics routines and some of Brian's medleys. He had no problem adjusting to the weights and started performing simple arm movements for approximately 30 minutes at Random Level 6. We didn't have to fight to keep him on the bike this time. He discovered that MuscleAerobics eased his boredom and "kept him occupied" while he rode the stationary bike.

Once he got "into the swing of things," he averaged 40 minutes at Random Level 6 per workout using a variety of lateral and arm swinging movements. He rarely varied his time, intensity level or arm movements. Because of his "routine" routine, he gave us a fairly consistent case study.

His recovery rate at the beginning of the study was approximately seven minutes. At the end of the study, he was recovering within two minutes. Craig did not report any weight change, but at the end of the study he was able to reach his target heart rate within four minutes, an 11-minute improvement!

Conclusion—When asked what he liked about MuscleAerobics and if he noticed any significant changes, he replied, "My body seemed to have had a better cardiovascular workout."

OUR HOPES FOR YOU

We think that you will come to the same conclusions we did about MuscleAerobics. We heartily encourage you to find out what it can do for you. Give yourself at least six weeks as a starting goal and be sure to use the form we've provided at the end of this chapter to keep records of your progress. We would love to hear about your MuscleAerobic experiences. Please mail your comments to: PaVàge Fitness, 200 E. Culver Boulevard, Playa del Rey, CA 90291.

Happy Fitness and welcome to MuscleAerobics!

MuscleAerobics Workout Form

Date: _____ Personal Body Weight: _____

Resting Heart Rate (RHR): _____ (Beats per minute while sitting)

Maximum Heart Rate (MHR): _____ (220 – your age)

Target Heart Rate (THR): _____ (60% to 80% x MHR)

Workout Day (Circle): M T W Th F St S

MuscleAerobics Program: _____ Aerobics Class _____ Stationary Bicycle

Amount Of Weight Used: _____ lbs. Duration Of Program: _____ min.

Aerobics Class Level*: _____ Stationary Bike Level**: _____

Time To Reach Target Heart Rate (THR): _____ min.

Time To Reach Recovery Rate (RR): _____ min.

General Comments: _____

_____

_____

_____

Date: _____ Personal Body Weight: _____

Resting Heart Rate (RHR): _____ (Beats per minute while sitting)

Maximum Heart Rate (MHR): _____ (220 – your age)

Target Heart Rate (THR): _____ (60% to 80% x MHR)

Workout Day (Circle): M T W Th F St S

MuscleAerobics Program: _____ Aerobics Class _____ Stationary Bicycle

Amount Of Weight Used: _____ lbs. Duration Of Program: _____ min.

Aerobics Class Level*: _____ Stationary Bike Level**: _____

Time To Reach Target Heart Rate (THR): _____ min.

Time To Reach Recovery Rate (RR): _____ min.

General Comments: _____

_____

_____

_____

* B=Beginning; I=Intermediate; A=Advanced
** Range of Difficulty from 1 (easiest) to 10 (most difficult)
If available, indicate random, interval or manual ride.

Weekly Progress Summary

	Initial	Goal	WEEKS									Total Change	Met Goal	Improved	No Change	Negative Gain
			2	4	6	8	10	12	14	16					
Weight															
Upper Arm															
Abdomen															
Waist															
Hips															
Thigh															
Calf															
Bust/Chest															
Skin Fold															
Biceps															
Triceps															
Iliac															

MuscleAerobics Survey

Age: _____ Occupation: _____ Sex: _____

City and state of residence: _____

Fitness/Sports activities you regularly engage in:

_____

_____

How long have you been doing MuscleAerobics? _____

Which MuscleAerobics program do you prefer and how much time do you
    spend on the program per session?
        Aerobics classes, Time: _____   Stationary bike, Time: _____

How do you like your MuscleAerobics program?
    Very Much _____   Like It _____   Don't Like It _____   Other _____

What type of benefits do you get from MuscleAerobics?
    Weight Loss _____
    Increased Endurance _____
    Greater Strength _____
    More Proportioned Physique _____
    Greater Muscular Endurance _____
    Better Overall Workout _____
    Other _____

What amount of weight do you use regularly? _____ lbs.

What brand of weights? _____

Have you discovered other benefits of MuscleAerobics that we have not
    mentioned in this book? If so, what are they?

_____

_____

In general, what do you think of MuscleAerobics?

_____

_____

Other comments:

_____

_____

Please mail to: MuscleAerobics
                c/o PaVage Fitness
                200 E. Culver Boulevard
                Playa del Rey, CA 90291

Acknowledgments

This book was possible due to the generous assistance of many people and organizations:

- Fuji Film U.S.A., Inc. for cooperation and superb photographic help. Special thanks to Carl Chapman and also Tim Mathiesen, our patient photographer.
- AMF Heavyhands for sponsorship support and for providing Heavyhands and stationary bicycles used in the book. Special thanks to Matt Dingman, Neil Talwar, Joyce Durlam and Phyllis.
- Reebok U.S.A. Limited, Inc. for sponsorship support and for providing the shoes and clothing worn by the models. Special thanks to Sharon Cohen, Angel Martinez, Jim Van Dine and Cathy Castles.
- For use of props thanks to Easton Aluminum, Bell Helmets, Weider Fitness Products and Mary-Mac Inc.
- For always coming to our last-minute needs, heartfelt thanks to Vicki Dooling of Designer Sports who provided men's clothing. Thank you Marc Valerio for the hats we used. For giving the crew plenty of figs to munch on, thanks to the California Fig Advisory Board. And for all the mineral water we could drink, thanks to Perrier.
- All of our great models were courtesy of PaVàge Fitness Images, 200 E. Culver Blvd., Playa del Rey, CA 90291. Special thanks to Erik Harden and Jeff Fink for helping us at the last minute.
- For expert advice and assistance on the medical and physiological aspects of MuscleAerobics, thanks to the Aerobics and Fitness Association of America, National Injury Prevention Foundation, David Pevsner, Jacqueline Ross, Dr. Leonard Schwartz and Linda Shelton. In addition, our gratitude to York Barbell, research librarians at University of California, Los Angeles and California State University, Northridge for helping us find the information we needed.
- For those who endured MuscleAerobics case studies, thanks to Brian, Craig, Vicki Andersen, Brett Costin, Mark Parigon and Tracy Leenley. We're sorry that space didn't permit everyone's story to be told! Special thanks to Karen Bauer, Vera Brown, Catherine Cassidy, Sheila Cluff, Lorna and Peter Francis, Linda and Dick Garton, Kym Hall, Rafer Johnson, Dale Lawlor, Phyllis McKenzie, Patrick Netter, Grace Olen, Siun Park, Nancy Petersen, Robert Miles Runyan, John Sammis, Barry Sanders, Esq., Ben Thomas and Jane Waldman.
- For confidence and support, thanks to our loving family: The Patano Crew—Mary and Chip, Ben, Stacy, Sarah, Nancy and Joan. The Savage Tribe—Sandy and Wayne, Amy, Thomas, Lindsay, JoAnne and Ron, Bert, Kathy, John, Loretta, Carlotta and Chuck.
- We must also thank the first MuscleAerobics participants of Linette's 6:15 a.m. aerobics class at Nautilus Plus in Encino, California. Gratitude to the Mid-Valley Athletic Club in Reseda, California for helping us to stay in shape.

Index

METRIC EQUIVALENTS

lbs.	gms
0.5	227
1.0	454
1.5	682
2.0	909
3.0	1363
4.0	1818
5.0	2272